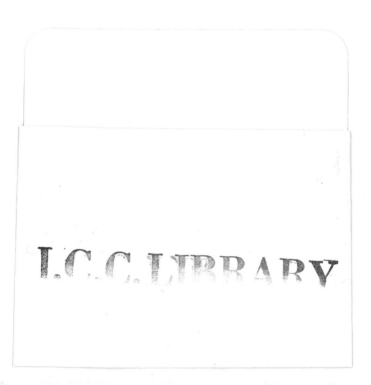

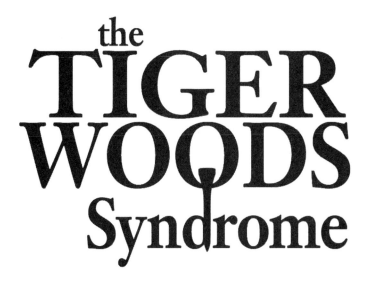

the TIGER WOODS Syndrome

*Why Men Prowl and
How to Not Become the Prey*

Dr. J. R. Bruns
Dr. R. A. Richards II

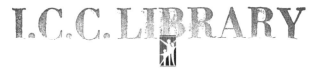

Health Communications, Inc.
Deerfield Beach, Florida

www.hcibooks.com

HQ
801
.B8738
.2010

Disclaimer: None of the people mentioned in this book have authorized or endorsed this book. The names and identifying information in this book have been changed to protect the privacy of the individuals and some details have been combined to create composite stories.

Library of Congress Cataloging-in-Publication Data
is available through the Library of Congress.

©Dr. J. R. Bruns and Dr. R. A. Richards II
ISBN-13: 978-0-7573-1537-4
ISBN-10: 0-7573-1537-2

Publisher: Health Communications, Inc.
        3201 S.W. 15th Street
        Deerfield Beach, FL 33442–8190

Cover photo ©Getty Images
Cover design by Larissa Hise Henoch
Interior design and formatting by Lawna Patterson Oldfield

To Jeanne, my wife.
Together we learned to live,
Share hope,
And experience joy.

♥♥♥ CONTENTS ♥♥♥

Part Two: Recovery and the Mirage Man

ACKNOWLEDGMENTS

The authors wish to thank Eddie Kritzer, who had the foresight to stick with us and help us develop the theme which became the name of this book.

His experience in publishing and knowing who to call helped us find the best publisher. We wish to thank all, and we hope readers will learn from this book, and be able to recognize the Tiger Woods Syndrome in their relationships.

"MEN HATE THOSE TO WHOM THEY HAVE TO LIE."

—*Victor Hugo (1802-1885)*

INTRODUCTION:
CATCHING A TIGER BY THE TAIL

*T*he *primary social unit* of our country is in a crisis. From the Oval Office on down, American marriages have been crumbling for decades. Illegitimacy and divorce are threatening the once solid bedrock of society. Sadly, few are immune from this destructive pattern. Religious people experience similar divorce rates as the unchurched. In every town across our country: cultural, athletic, moral, education, and political leaders are falling almost daily to personal scandal, the result of failed marriages. Politicians look to correct the symptoms, but no one has correctly identified the reason for the decline of the American family.

When the fairy-tale world of Tiger Woods came crashing down on Thanksgiving, it caused Americans to pause from their holiday reverie and wonder how someone who had it all could lead such a double life, cheating not just once but in a serial fashion. Yet this is not some aberration. We—psychiatrist Dr. J. R. Bruns and Dr. R. A. Richards— have studied men leading dual lives just like Tiger Woods, from celebrities to the average guy in the barber shop. We have identified a distinct pattern of duplicitous male behavior and named it the Tiger Woods Syndrome because Tiger so aptly exemplifies the behaviors, motivations, and destructive patterns of so many American men.

This is the first book to identify the Tiger Woods Syndrome: a five-stage pattern of dating and mating behavior that has resulted in untold suffering by millions of shattered families. We will introduce you to this increasingly common malady that begins with two lovers head over heels for each other and ends with two bitterly disappointed and estranged partners, often headed to divorce court.

The root of the Tiger Woods Syndrome is the artificial way men and women relate to one another as they try to find a common life together. We will show how prevalent this failed method of relating has become in America over the last century and how it presents itself in day-to-day behavior, whether you are on your second date or preparing to walk down the aisle. The good news is that this disorder can be corrected. It is possible for men and women to replace artificial intimacy with authenticity and to rebuild a solid foundation and a healthier way of being together. By applying the advice in the second half of the book, you can heal your relationship and make it a positive example for the next generation. A fulfilling relationship based on honesty is indeed possible—and we will illuminate a path to help you find it.

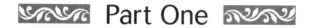 Part One

ASSESSING ROMANTIC RELATIONSHIPS TODAY

1

SAY IT AIN'T SO!

"My wife, we're in it together.
We're a team, and we do things as a team.
And I care about her with all my heart."

—*Tiger Woods, September 21, 2006*

*P*rofessional golfer Tiger Woods was one of the greatest American sports heroes in history. He stepped into our consciousness as a two-year-old on the *Mike Douglas Show*, hitting a golf ball under the careful tutelage of his father, Earl. He dominated the high school and college golf world, and, upon turning pro, won seventy-one Professional Golfers' Association (PGA) tournaments, including fourteen major golf championships. He has earned almost a billion dollars in prize money and endorsements.

Tiger's success piqued interest both within and outside of the world of golf, and even people who weren't sports fans took notice of this extremely talented athlete. He was named the Associated Press Athlete of the Year and *Sports Illustrated* Sportsman of the Year. He hobnobbed with Oprah Winfrey, Roger Federer, and Michael Jordan. He addressed the nation at "We Are One: The Obama Inaugural Celebration at the Lincoln Memorial" and visited the White House in April

2009. He established numerous youth charity projects, including the Start Something character development program, the Tiger Woods Foundation, In the City golf clinics and festivals, and the Tiger Woods Learning Center. With his polyglot ancestry and globe-trotting golf schedule, he was a role model to billions and the most recognizable sports celebrity in the world. In 2004, Tiger wed the Swedish beauty Elin Nordegren, and several years later Elin gave birth to two children (a girl in 2007 and a boy in 2009). Tiger had love, family, success, fame, and fortune. What more could a man desire?

The fairy-tale life of Tiger Woods came crashing down Thanksgiving night 2009. Sketchy cable news reports said that Tiger had been in a one-vehicle accident and had gone to the hospital. Tabloids soon published lurid charges of a domestic disturbance. On December 2, 2009, the worst fears of the worldwide public were realized when Tiger issued a terse apology for "personal failings" and "transgressions."

The first question on the minds of the world was "Why?" Why throw away a life of success and respect for a series of meaningless flings with cocktail waitresses, prostitutes, and pornography starlets? How could the idol of millions appear to be so wholesome and yet live a secret double life of shame?

Was the Tiger Woods we had all known and loved a man or a mirage?

Unfortunately, Tiger Woods is not the exception. Many have coined 2009 as the Year of the Cad. *Late Show* host David Letterman admitted to a series of covert relationships with his female staffers and personal assistant, turning the historic Ed Sullivan Theater into his own fraternity house. John Edwards, 2004 vice presidential candidate, revealed a long-rumored liaison with a videographer while his terminally ill wife was out campaigning for him. Former NFL quarterback Steve McNair was murdered by a jilted lover while his unassuming wife and children lived in another state. South Carolina governor Mark Sanford disappeared for a week to rendezvous with an Argentine lover, and disgraced former New York governor Eliot Spitzer attempted to return to public life only months after being caught in a sting operation on the swanky Emperor's Club call girl's ring.

Tiger, Dave, John, Steve, Mark, and Eliot all crafted an image of successful family men but turned out to be mirages to those who loved them most and thought they knew them best. Sadly, this reprehensible behavior isn't limited to just the rich and famous. This same deceptive behavior is just as common in the heartland as the cities, and is practiced by the clerk taking your money at the local Gas-N-Sip and the middle-class guy struggling to make a living with two kids and a mortgage in the suburbs. With millions of American males embracing the values of Tiger Woods, how can American women possibly avoid being snookered by such love frauds?

This book has good news for all those hoping to avoid the fate of Elin Nordegren. We can learn from Tiger's mistakes. A fulfilling relationship based on honesty is possible. The secret to a happy relationship is staring us in the face, but we need to adopt an activist stance. First, we need to examine our life histories and past relationships. Think back to the days of your innocent school-yard crushes, high school flames, prom dates, college romances, steady boyfriends/girlfriends, and your marriage. Consider how they started, how they progressed, and how they ended (if they did). Were there patterns to the mating dance? How did you behave when you first met and during the romance? Now examine how you reacted as the relationship expired. Do you see a rhythm to the ritual?

The Bill Murray movie *Groundhog Day* featured this notion of repeating patterns in relationships. Bill Murray played Phil, a smart-aleck TV weatherman for a small-market station. On February 2, the TV station sends Phil to Punxsutawney, Pennsylvania, to cover the annual

Groundhog Day festivities with his estranged producer Rita (played by the lovely Andie MacDowell). Something changes in the universe and Phil is forced to relive February 2 over and over, like an episode of *The Twilight Zone*. Phil eventually learns to use this opportunity to change his interests, skills, beliefs, and goals to conform to Rita's and gradually wins her heart. Once Phil becomes Rita's dream guy, the repetitive curse is lifted.

Think about the manner in which Phil goes about winning Rita. In the movie Phil and Rita end up living happily ever after, but in real life would this relationship last? Phil only changed to win Rita. He didn't go into therapy to find out why he lived his entire life as a selfish, egotistical, miserable human being.

Those who give up smoking or drinking find out how hard it is to truly change even a small part of one's behavior. Now think about how hard it would be to change every part of your life—every taste, every natural impulse, every habit. Through the intervention of the fate, Phil manages to do it as a short-term goal to gain the hand of Rita. Once Phil achieves his goal and loses his motivation to change, wouldn't it be likely he would revert back to his bad old self? In *Groundhog II* wouldn't we be more likely to see an unshaven

Phil lying on the couch in his T-shirt and sweat bottoms, watching sports and barking orders for another beer from the snookered Rita?

The exaggerated patterns of *Groundhog Day* are instructive in understanding why marriages in America are so unfulfilling. Men just like Tiger seek superficial conformity to their lady's tastes to conjure up the familiar spirits of intimacy. Later, when the thrill of the romance fades, the woman is often stuck with a stranger. How many times has this pattern happened to you, women readers? If you are a man, how many times did you hide your true self from the woman you were dating?

More and more women are finding themselves stuck with cranky strangers. *Los Angeles Times* columnist Robin Abcarian describes a telling account of three working mothers checking in with each other in an article entitled "Happily Married . . . or Just Nuts?":

❖

Wife 1, cautiously: Do you ever feel like your husband just doesn't like you?

Wife 2: All the time!

Wife 3: It's one of my standard fighting refrains: "If you dislike me so much, why did you ever marry me?"

Wife 1: When I ask other friends about this, they all look at me like I'm crazy, like they don't know what I'm talking about.

Wife 1 and Wife 2, in unison: Liars, liars, pants on fire.[1]

How often have you heard a female friend complaining about her spouse, describing a litany of obnoxious traits and a grumpy disposition? Then, when asked why she ever married such a boorish lout, her response is, "Well, Frank was nothing like this when we were dating."

Women readers, that is the key to understanding men. Many men are not their true selves when they are dating you—they are mirages. Like Tiger Woods, many American men seek superficial values, hide their true feelings, and conform to win their dream girls. Commercials, television shows, movies, and even music drum into men's brains that conformity and deception are part of the dating and mating scene.

Now that we know what is wrong with relationships from the outset, what can we do to stop repeating the failed dating game over and over in our own private *Groundhog Day*?

To achieve a satisfying relationship, women must learn to recognize these smooth-talking love salesmen. Men must unlearn this harmful pattern so they can stop this insane method of courtship and marriage. By studying the concepts in the following chapters, both male and female readers will learn healthy ways of relating to the opposite sex and hopefully avoid the pain and broken dreams of Tiger and Elin Nordegren.

2

ARE YOU IN AN UNHEALTHY RELATIONSHIP?

*M*any people know their friends and family have unhealthy relationships but are not able to see that the same may apply to their own romance or marriage. This short quiz will help you cut through the fog to see if your past or present unions are unhealthy and in need of improvement.

1. How long did you know the person before you first dated them?
    a. More than one year.
    b. More than one month.
    c. Less than one month.

2. How long did you date your significant other before you first kissed them?
    a. One date.
    b. Two to three dates.
    c. Four or more dates.

3. How long did you date your significant other before you first became physically intimate?
    a. Less than one month.

b. More than one month but less than six months.

c. More than six months.

4. On the date(s) before you became physically intimate, did you keep things superficial, or did you mutually share your attitudes, interests, and goals?

a. Mutually shared our attitudes, interests, and goals.

b. Started superficially but eventually shared our attitudes, interests, and goals.

c. Kept things superficial.

5. How soon after you first began dating did you become engaged?

a. Within six months of our first date.

b. Between six months and a year of our first date.

c. More than one year after our first date.

6. How soon after you first began dating did you move in together?

a. More than one year after our first date.

b. Between six months and a year after our first date.

c. Within six months after our first date.

7. When you began dating, how much did you share in common?

a. We had many similar attitudes, interests, and goals.

b. We had some similar attitudes, interests, and goals.

c. We had few if any common attitudes, interests, and goals.

8. Would you describe your dating as more time spent at romantic dinners, movies, dances, and nightclubs, or in

slowly getting to know each other in mostly nonromantic settings?

   a. Our dating was mostly romantic dinners, movies, dances, and nightclubs.

   b. Our dating was a mix of romantic activities and nonromantic time spent getting to know each other.

   c. Our dating was primarily spent in nonromantic settings getting to know each other.

9. If, before you ever met, it was determined that you could never be in a physical relationship with your significant other, would you now be:

   a. Close friends.

   b. Acquaintances.

   c. Strangers.

10. Do you generally do the things you used to enjoy before your present relationship began?

   a. I rarely do the things I used to enjoy before our relationship began.

   b. I occasionally do the things I used to enjoy before our relationship began.

   c. I generally have continued to do the things I enjoyed doing before our relationship began.

11. Did you have to go through a severe emotional crisis (possibly including infidelity and/or separation) before establishing a stable, enduring relationship?

   a. No crisis to a moderate adjustment period once we began living together.

b. Major crisis that threatened the relationship.

c. Infidelity/trial separation/divorce and remarriage.

12. Do you and your significant other currently share activities and interests besides family obligations?

   a. Few if any.

   b. Some activities and interests.

   c. Many activities and interests.

13. Do you and your significant other conduct separate lives outside the home?

   a. Aside from work and family obligations, we spend most of our free time together.

   b. Aside from work and family obligations, we spend some free time together and some with friends.

   c. Aside from work and family obligations, we spend little time together.

14. Do you feel free to share your feelings with your significant other?

   a. No. Are you kidding? I don't want to make him/her upset.

   b. Sometimes, depending on the situation.

   c. Yes.

Points for each answer: 3 for an unhealthy response, 2 for somewhat unhealthy, 1 for healthy.

ANSWER KEY

1. A. **1**   B. **2**   C. **3**

2. A. **3**   B. **2**   C. **1**

3. A. **3**   B. **2**   C. **1**

4. A. **1**   B. **2**   C. **3**

5. A. **3**   B. **2**   C. **1**

6. A. **1**   B. **2**   C. **3**

7. A. **1**   B. **2**   C. **3**

8. A. **3**   B. **2**   C. **1**

9. A. **1**   B. **2**   C. **3**

10. A. **3**   B. **2**   C. **1**

11. A. **1**   B. **2**   C. **3**

12. A. **3**   B. **2**   C. **1**

13. A. **3**   B. **1**   C. **2**

14. A. **3**   B. **2**   C. **1**

Points 14–21: You have a generally healthy relationship. This book will encourage you to keep doing the right things to keep the momentum going. Well done.

Points 22–31: Caution: Your relationship has potential deception and superficial experiences at its core. You could be headed for eventual heartbreak. Read this book and be alert for the danger signs and how to remedy them to make your relationship more complete.

Points 32–42: Danger! The warning signs suggest that you are in a relationship based on deceit. Hopefully by reading this book you can find help and healing if you want it.

3

LOVE AMERICAN STYLE: COURTSHIP AND MARRIAGE

"History teaches us that man learns nothing from history."

—*Georg Wilhelm Friedrich Hegel, philosopher*

*D*uring *the early research* for this book, we were charting the behavior of the mirage man but had not yet condensed it into a predictable pattern of human behavior. Most of the foibles of these deceivers were mocked in the daily comic strips as diverse as *Adam, For Better Or For Worse,* and *Hagar the Horrible.* Growing up in a culture that was steeped in superficiality, it was assumed that this had always been the way men and women courted and married.

It was, needless to say, a shock to find out that our grade school, high school, and college history courses had neglected to touch on the profound changes in courtship and marriage. We discovered there was a historical basis to the sick behavior afflicting modern couples. It must be understood to deal with the Tiger Woods Syndrome.

Love and marriage changed dramatically over America's 234 years of existence. Our colonial model of courtship and matrimony was initially based on the host nations of our founding fathers and mothers. The predominately Western European immigrant marriage of the colonial period was largely determined by ethnicity, class, and creed. As in the Old Country, marriage was often an economic merger of families.

The strange new political experiment of democracy in the New World touched all aspects of life. The Age of Enlightenment demanded that all things must be questioned and reformed, including the way American men and women found a new life together.

Harvard University professor Werner Sollors noted this radical change in the hearts and minds of the upstart colonists. Americans embraced the idea that the nobility and rigid classes that separated one citizen from another were just another oppressive system from Europe. Just as all men were created equal, then all men should be equal in courtship and marriage. It followed that consent, not descent, should determine romantic relationships just as consent determined citizenship after the American Revolution. Thus, romantic love became a requirement for marriage just as love of country became a prerequisite of American citizenship.

This landmark change in courtship and marriage took generations to spread throughout the fledgling democracy.

Ethnicity, class, and religion—as well as the dangerous concepts of free choice and romantic love— formed an amalgam that guided early post–Revolutionary War American decisions on love and matrimony. Professor Sollors documented this evolving new freedom in romance by such fascinated impartial observers as nineteenth-century French critic Alexis de Tocqueville, who spread this new idea of choice to Europe.

Initially, there was fierce resistance to the idea of basing a marriage on the ephemeral notion of "falling in love." But prominent nineteenth-century Anglo-American intellectuals such as Lord Byron and Robert and Elizabeth Barrett Browning popularized the idea of romantic love in poetry and literature. By the mid-1800s, the American culture embraced romantic love as "the key to domestic harmony rather than a threat to it."[1]

By the Gay 90s, courtship had changed significantly. Books and plays recounting that era described dates "away from home, unchaperoned, and not subject to parental veto."[2] By the dawn of the twentieth century, the arranged ethnic, religious, and class courtship of first-generation Americans arriving at our shores was giving way to the strange new American courtship of unsupervised free will.

While the choice of a marriage partner had become an

exercise of free will for nineteenth-century Americans, Alexis de Tocqueville noted in his 1840 work, *Democracy in America* that the independence of American women "is irrevocably lost in the bonds of matrimony."[3] This was due to the patriarchal structure of American marriages. They emphasized rigid roles that each partner would fulfill, regardless of romantic feelings, to achieve the common goal of economic success and the perpetuation of the family through the generations by procreation.[4] While romantic love came to be thought essential to the selection of the marriage partner, these euphoric feelings of courtship enjoyed by the woman were eclipsed by the overwhelming burden of almost immediate and extended motherhood.[5]

In the early part of the twentieth century, the patriarchal system underwent an American revolution. During this era of suffragette/feminist intellectual thought and the eventual granting of the right to vote in elections, the new companionate marriage model emerged.

In sharp contrast to the patriarchal model, the companionate marriage emphasized men and women as coequals. Romantic love was not only necessary during courtship as in the American-style patriarchal model, but it was mandatory to keep two equal partners together after the wedding

ceremony. In a radical shift from the patriarchal model, a fulfilling sexual relationship was required during the life of the
companionate marriage. With no defined roles to follow,
daily communication was key in delegating duties among
equals, including child rearing.[6]

The old stereotypical roles that guided American couples
through marriage were now deemed old-fashioned and
oppressive. Beginning with the intellectual elite and celebrities, this marriage reform was slowly but surely embraced by
middle America. The successful experiment of female
employment in businesses and factories during World War
II, as well as female service in the armed forces, convinced
millions of men that the companionate model made sense.

By the 1950s American women were beginning to retain
the freedom in marriage that they had enjoyed in courtship.
American youth culture practiced a new way of determining
male compatibility for future brides in coequal marriages
through the custom of "going steady." Dates were used to
demonstrate that the man could satisfy his partner's romantic needs.[7]

The American institution was shaken to its foundation by
this contemporary concept of coupledom. By the mid-twentieth
century, romance—not economic success and dynastic pro-

gression—was considered essential in marriage. Historian Jeffrey Weeks observed that at this point in time American marriage was "no longer the permanent bond it was intended to be."[8]

The 1960s lawmakers followed this marriage revolution with sweeping legal changes. Soon such restrictions as grounds for divorce were legislated away as old-fashioned and unfair. Syndicated writer Mona Charen observed these legal reforms were based on the companionate assumption that if "marriage isn't making both partners happy, why not permit divorce?"[9]

Millions have abandoned ship on their sinking marriages since these lax divorce laws have come into existence. Unfortunately, both partners are often unable to give their spouse what they yearn for in a companionate marriage because the requirements are so subjective. Whereas a patriarchal husband merely had to "bring home the bacon" and his wife attend to her considerable duties to satisfy the letter of the marriage, companionate unions require such ethereal notions as "intimacy, companionship, someone to understand us and be a soul mate."[10] Once the ephemeral emotional high of a relationship fades, there is little in the eye of the beholder to keep the couple together. All that remains of these spent unions is attorney services, court dates, and the endless search for the relational Holy Grail.

A key weakness in the companionate model of courtship and marriage is the requirement of honesty. If both partners are candid in their courtship, there is a strong possibility they will chose to marry based on a full disclosure of the strengths and weaknesses of each partner. As coequals, negotiations and allowances will be made before irreversible commitment to the diversity of both partners so their individuality won't be smothered in the marriage union. Neither will feel defrauded after marriage by the reasonable behavior of one another.

COURTSHIP, MARRIAGE, AND THE SLIPPERY SLOPE

Historian Ellen K. Rothman's exhaustive study of nineteenth-century American middle-class courtship and marriage, entitled *Hands and Hearts: A History of Courtship in America*, reports that marriage in America was once predicated on honest courtship. When America was a rural land, boys and girls grew up together and selected their mates from a pool of acquaintances they had often known since birth. The superficial qualities of looks and charm were less important than one's character and shared interests. Couples thus relied on open communication to protect against the twin plagues of "insincerity and misplaced affections."[11]

Rothman has documented the sad, slow slide of nineteenth-century healthy courtship and marriage into what we now call the Tiger Woods Syndrome. Beginning after the Civil War, America became increasingly urban, with many migrating to the cities for employment in nonagrarian industries. Concurrently, more young men and women began attending colleges. Technology, such as the bicycle, car, and telephone, increased the size of the once-small American village. These various trends of the Industrial Revolution from 1870 to the 1920s had one significant result on relationships: Americans began living among strangers and soon began courting and marrying them.[12]

❖

At first, American men and women resisted the call to abandon the tried-and-true courtship values of character and communication. However, a strong and persuasive mass media soon began to plant doubts in the generations coming of age, with the damning argument that healthy dating was "old-fashioned."[13] The new courtship emphasized physical attraction and charm and inhibited candor and openness. It was a siren song of destruction for our once-strong American marriages.

In the early to mid-twentieth century, healthy courtship that emphasized the sharing of confidences was being phased out in favor of this new courtship of "catching a mate," while at the same time, the model of American marriage was also changing from patriarchal to companionate. The table starting on page 30 illustrates the results of old-fashioned healthy and unhealthy "catch-a-mate" courtship based on both the old-fashioned patriarchal and modern companionate marriage models.

As the table shows, the results of the companionate marriage model are extremely poor if the marriage is founded on the sandy bedrock of dishonest courtship. Parents, educators, and the media are not instructing American sons and daughters of this stringent requirement of full disclosure in dating before committing to one another. The result is a mutation of the companionate model of courtship and marriage into the Tiger Woods Syndrome, resulting in a plague of unstable marriages that threatens our very society.

How did this mutation occur? Growing numbers of young men, largely instructed by their ignorant peers and heavily influenced by the media of music, film, and later television, learned to cheat the system. If contemporary courtship success is based upon sexual attraction and suitability as lovers, then pretending to be emotionally compatible would greatly increase the chances of positive short-term courtship results. In an American society that praises the concept of living for the moment, deceivers are the winners. The Tiger Woods Syndrome is defined as men defrauding women for immediate companionship. It has become an accepted way of life for many American men.

As we can see from the chart comparing patriarchal versus companionate marriage, American men learned there is no need for lifetime compatibility in the companionate marriage model as it has the inherent weakness of the subjective value of self-fulfillment. Aided by their mostly male legislators that have lessened the sting of divorce, men have realized that marriages are as easy to dissolve as a commercial contract. Today, American men are recklessly pursuing marriage as a short-term goal. If it doesn't work out, no hard feelings!

Historically, society has condoned this selfish male behavior. Singer/actor Frank Sinatra's famous 1950s comeback as a

Types of Marriage Models

Companionate Marriage

HEALTHY COURTSHIP

1. Both partners would experience a mutually satisfying, personally fulfilling romantic relationship.
2. No defined duties; roles would vary or would be negotiated between both partners.
3. Due to honest basis of relationship there would be no peak (honeymoon) and the inevitable disillusionment after the honeymoon fades.
4. Marriage would be marked by true intimacy between partners.
5. Relationship would as a byproduct fulfill the patriarchal goal of perpetuation of the family through the generations if both partners agree to it during their initial courtship.
6. Economic success would be achieved by both partners or either partner choosing to be in the role of "breadwinner." The success of the relationship would eliminate the economically debilitating effect of divorce/alimony/child support.
7. Relationship is based on a day-to-day romantic relationship over duty. Both partners would expect it throughout the marriage.

ARTIFICIAL INTIMACY

1. The wife is cheated out of a personally fulfilling romantic relationship by her dishonest husband who deceived her to begin the relationship.
2. The marriage lacks true intimacy and depending on the stubbornness or psychological state of denial by the partners, tends to be short-lived.
3. The romantic aspect of the relationship ends once the wife realizes there is something wrong and begins diminishing sexual relations with the man. He responds by withdrawing romantically. His resentment increases at this point, and he begins to reveal his true self to his wife. Both partners end up completely miserable.
4. No defined duties, but the husband often resents the wife because he doesn't negotiate in an honest manner when the companionate style roles are discussed. He often secretly wants the marriage roles to be patriarchal but pretends to accept his wife's choice of the companionate marriage style. He may wait until the honeymoon is over to tell his shocked wife what he really expects her roles to be.
5. Patriarchal goals of perpetuation of the family unit by procreation and economic success are jeopardized by the ephemeral nature of the marriage. There is a high probability of divorce with its crippling economic effects and its destructive effects on the children, weakening their future resolve to continue the family line.

HEALTHY COURTSHIP

Patriarchal Marriage

1. The common goals of the patriarchal marriage would be agreed to by both partners before the relationship became committed. These are the perpetuation of the family unit through procreation and economic success through a predetermined division of labor by the husband and wife.
2. Rigid, well-defined roles would be willingly fulfilled by both partners without resentment.
3. True intimacy would be a feature of this marriage and would sustain the couple once the children have grown up and moved away.
4. No honeymoon peak period as both partners would be well-informed before committing to one another the expected roles each was to fulfill. Each would know the other person and would not face the inevitable post-honeymoon disillusion.

ARTIFICIAL INTIMACY

1. Both partners settle into a post-honeymoon, non-romantic relationship with only well-defined separate roles to fulfill (example, Joseph and Rose Kennedy's marriage.)
2. Due to the deceptive nature of the courtship, both partners may not share a common view on the patriarchal goals of the marriage and may become resentful and display addictive behavior as they numb their pain in their life-long commitment.
3. Rigid, well-defined roles are often unwillingly fulfilled as the partners seethe resentment and disappointment at each other.
4. The marriage lacks true intimacy but both partners remain committed to the marriage to fulfill the goals of perpetuation of the family unit through procreation and economic success of the family unit through a predetermined division of labor by the husband and wife.
5. There is no reason for the partners to pretend to care for each other once the children have grown up and left and both partners are economically secure. They will live out their waning years in estrangement from one another, sharing on a deep-seated mutual resentment of each other.

leader of the Rat Pack was embraced by the popular culture as hip and enlightened. Sinatra and his cronies made unhealthy courtship and weak companionate marriages the norm. After years of infidelity, Sinatra finally left his wife and kids for a tempestuous relationship with Ava Gardner and later impulsively married a young actress named Mia Farrow who was decades younger. This cheapening of marriage by cultural icons like the men in the Rat Pack had a long-term deleterious effect on America. Fellow Rat Packers like Dean Martin and Sammy Davis Jr. "shook up the idea that American males should be stoic, monogamous good providers."[14] That "stoic" stability of the male was the upside of patriarchal marriages, and it should have been carried over to the new companionate marriages.

Beginning in earnest in the 1950s and becoming the prevalent view in the 1960s and 1970s, movies, music, and television conferred heroic status on the prowling, transient male who can only stay a while, because his greater calling is to "follow the sun" or some other excuse for abandoning his wife and family once he no longer feels personally fulfilled. Barbara Dafoe Whitehead, a recognized authority on American marriage, agrees that "we just aren't holding men accountable for bad behavior" anymore.[15]

The metamorphosis of romance did not stop with this new form of deceitful companionate marriage. With societal mores on illegitimacy and premarital sex falling to the wayside in the psychedelic 1960s and the "me generation" in the 1970s, marriage itself could be avoided. From 1970 to 1995, cohabitating unmarried couples increased more than 700 percent.[16] Why? American men and women realized that the new style of dishonest courtship led to such unstable relationships that it was foolish to invest the time, emotional capital, legal entanglements, and money to get married. It became obvious to the average person that marriage success had decreased to a coin flip.

Belief in the success of marriage now requires a faith reserved for religion in times past. Thus, cohabitation and serial monogamy are at an all-time high. People are applying the mutated companionate courtship values of sexual attraction and contrived compatibility in choosing cohabitation partners. In an interview with television and movie star George Clooney on his 1980s decision to move in with actress Kelly Preston on their first date, Clooney concluded, "I was always Mr. Full-On Spontaneous . . . then as you get older, you start to go, 'You know what? Maybe we should go out a little bit first'."[17] What—go out and get to know each other before moving in together? For many mirage men that is an unthinkable idea. But the results of this deceitful cohabitation trend have been anything but encouraging, with a break-up rate for couples who cohabitate twice as high as for married couples.[18] Washington State University researcher Jan Stets reported that women who cohabitate are more than twice as likely to be victims of domestic violence than married women and data from the National Institute of Mental Health show that cohabitating women have three times the rate of depression as married women and twice as much as non-cohabitating single women.[19]

Why isn't cohabitation working? The problem is that the male partner is often pretending to be emotionally compatible to achieve immediate sexual results and uses cohabitation to subvert the dating process altogether.[20] By living together, the female partner often sees the real man behind the phony act and realizes she has been deceived by her man way before marriage. Thus, any cohabitation that limps into marriage is already weakened before the wedding ceremony by the already jaded bride.

An example of this crippled cohabitation is found in legendary *Late Show* host David Letterman, who used to joke regularly about the polar relationship he endured with his twenty-year live-in girlfriend before he married her in March 2009. Yet that low level of happiness was long before Letterman's wife discovered he was having multiple sexual relationships with staffers at work. We can only imagine the subzero atmosphere at Dave's ranch in Montana inside the main house in the middle of July.

Whether in cohabitation or marriage, healthy relationships between women and men are at an all-time low. The sad result of the decline in heterosexual relations in the last century is that today, in the new millennium, college women are faced with an all-or-nothing choice in relationships. The customs of even twenty years ago—when coeds would meet men, become friends, date, and only then become committed to each other in a monogamous relationship—no longer exist.[21]

HOOKING UP OR JOINED AT THE HIP

The landmark study Hooking Up, Hanging Out and Hoping for Mr. Right, commissioned and funded by the Independent Women's Focus and released by the Institute for American Values, reported that women in modern America are given the choice of two extreme models of romantic heterosexual relationships: "hooking up" or being "joined at the hip." The hookup, practiced by 40 percent of women in the study, is "friends with benefits," meaning casual sex without commitment. The other common relationship is joined at the hip, where a couple that doesn't know each other very well commits to a sexual relationship and spends all their time together.

The authors of the study, University of Texas sociology professor Norval Glenn and associate scholar with the Institute for American Values, Elizabeth Marquardt, concluded that neither hooking up nor being joined at the hip is likely to lead college women to their goal of an intelligent, long-term, committed relationship that might lead to marriage.[22] Yet the hookup and being joined at the hip are custom-made for the deceitful man who wants immediate gratification.

Time after time women mistakenly think they have found their soul mates, but they are continually astonished to discover it was just another mirage. Whether they are hooking up, joined at the hip, cohabitating, or marrying, women are cheated out of a fulfilling companionate relationship by the twenty-first-century scourge of romance: the "mirage men." This deceitful form of the companionate model of courtship and marriage is practiced by mirage men like Tiger Woods, John Edwards, Steve McNair, Mark Sanford, Eliot Spitzer, and David Letterman.

Now that we have examined the historical roots of the Tiger Woods Syndrome, let's examine two distinct types of mirage men, whose behavior causes exploitation and dissatisfaction for women—and heartbreak and misery for both partners.

4

THE TWO FACES OF
THE MIRAGE MAN

"God give me strength to face
a fact though it slay me."

—Thomas Huxley
English biologist (1825-1895)

*T**he goal of the mirage man* is to deceive women
to gain immediate companionship. This usually
begins with a deceptive form of courtship that attracts a
person who may or may not be compatible. Over time,
each relationship goes through five distinct stages in the
same order. These five stages are: (1) the allure of artificial
intimacy; (2) approval seeking; (3) commitment/
abandonment; (4) the honeymoon; and (5) resigned compliance. Each stage leads to more commitment by both partners,
binding them to an increasingly destructive relationship. In
Chapters 5 through 9, we will examine all five stages in detail
and instruct the reader in some helpful ways to make their
current relationship more complete. Reading the information in this book will help couples discern if their relationship reflects the tendencies of dysfunctional relationship
whether they are married or living together. By learning to
recognize the successive steps of this pattern, which leads to

a union of diminished intimacy, both men and women will be able to evaluate their commitment to each other and take the necessary steps to restore their relationships.

But before discussing each stage in detail, let's look at the two possible strains of mirage men: the misogynist mirage man and the compliant mirage man. Both types of men go through all five stages of the Tiger Woods Syndrome, but each may react to it differently. Let's look at each of these types in detail.

THE MISOGYNIST MIRAGE MAN

The misogynist mirage man has been well documented in Susan Forward's bestseller, *Men Who Hate Women and the Women Who Love Them*.[1] The misogynist has a Prince Charming personality before the relationship hits its emotional peak (the honeymoon period, or Stage 4 of the Tiger Woods Syndrome). He is willing to temporarily surrender control of the relationship to the woman to get companionship and sexual favors, but he enters the relationship with the mind-set of disrespect and bitterness at womankind. Into this cauldron of hatred is added the resentments accrued in the present relationship, which will be expressed once the thrill of the romance or marriage cools.

Ultimately, the prince transforms into a monstrous, foul-tempered frog once the rewards of companionship and sex lose their anesthetic potency and his personal demons can no longer be contained. Then it is the woman who must decide whether to live in a house of fear or leave this loaded pistol.

A good example of a classic misogynist mirage man is O. J. Simpson. A generation before Tiger Woods, he became the greatest college football player at the University of Southern California, and then achieved even greater stardom playing for the Buffalo Bills in the National Football League. Like Tiger, he exuded charisma and quickly bridged the gap between blacks and whites for an America emerging from a 100-year post–Civil War racial divide. "The Juice" became as familiar in commercials as the gridiron and later was an actor and a commentator on the extremely popular ABC-TV's *Monday Night Football.*

While the unsuspecting world adored him, O. J. Simpson led a dual life in the fast lane. His hatred of women resulted in repeated physical abuse of his second wife, Nicole Brown Simpson, and she was eventually murdered one balmy June night in tony Brentwood, California.

THE COMPLIANT MIRAGE MAN

The compliant mirage man is mentally capable of loving women but unfortunately uses deceit to gain a sexual relationship. He may be a "good" person, but he has bought into the predominant cultural view that the romantic ends justify the means. The results for this man, as we will see in detail in the following chapters, are quite ironic.

Despite healthy motives, the compliant mirage man eventually finds himself feeling as mentally resentful as the misogynist. Why? A tremendous resentment builds up in the compliant man. After the honeymoon peak of the relationship fades, the compliant man begins to tire of always accommodating his partner. She has no idea why his heart is no longer in the activities and events he seemed to enjoy so much with her during their early courtship. But the only way for him to preserve the relationship is to continue acceding to her wishes. Thus, he feels trapped. He eventually looks to his beloved as his oppressor and often begins to live a secret life, doing the things he really enjoys.

Tiger Woods's text message to Lover #1, Rachel Uchitel, indicates that he had reached this point in his compliant mirage man marriage when his dual life was exposed. He texted, "I know it's brutal on you that you can't be with me all the time. I get it. It [expletive deleted] kills me, too. I finally found someone I connect with."[2] In Tiger's case, he resented being married to Elin Nordegren and lived a secret life of risky sexual encounters.

There are two different outcomes for compliant mirage men. In "miserable" compliant mirage relationships, the woman eventually realizes that the man deceived her into thinking he was her Prince Charming and starts to detest the sniveling wimp who will do anything to please her. This is your classic henpecked husband.

In "happy" compliant mirage relationships, his mate may never discover his deception. If she does, she won't discover the mirage man's treachery until after he dies, a scandal is revealed (as in Tiger's case), or he finally snaps. She will be the last to know, even though his deceitful behavior may be well known in the community. The guy who cons a community out of their life savings and is finally exposed decades later usually is this type of compliant mirage man.

Although the misogynist and compliant mirage men have radically different marriages and cohabitations with women, they share the same five-stage pattern of development of their deceptive relationships and the same ultimate result:

both partners are cheated out of mutually satisfying and personally fulfilling companionate relationships. Thus, both are subclasses of the same scourge of love: the mirage man.

Mirage men have been with us since the fall in the Garden of Eden. There have always been deceivers who could take advantage of women who loved to have their ears tickled with flatteries. But society didn't condone it; it warned both men and women to beware of such scoundrels who promise much and deliver heartbreak. In the last century, film, television, and music did an about-face and began glorifying dishonest men and gullible women. Plays like *South Pacific, Guys and Dolls, West Side Story,* and *The Music Man* gradually turned public opinion from disgust to sympathy for the mirage man. Movies like *Casablanca, An Officer and a Gentleman, Witness, Sixteen Candles,* and *Titanic* made love at first sight seem desirable. Singers like Frank Sinatra, Jim Morrison, and Johnny Cash glorified the live-for-the-moment behavior of mirage men. Television shows like *Two and a Half Men, How I Met Your Mother, Seinfeld, Friends,* and *Everybody Loves Raymond* made artificial intimacy and approval seeking seem like the only way to have a relationship. To past generations, the notion of using deception to attain true love was fascinating because it was so unusual.

Thanks to a century of media promotion, deceit is now the culturally sanctioned way to romantic bliss. In Chapter 5, we will examine the first stop on the road to this unhealthy relationship: artificial intimacy.

5

GOT TO GET YOU INTO MY LIFE: STAGE 1— *ARTIFICIAL INTIMACY*

"People say certain things to each other.
'I love you!' 'You mean everything to me!'
Everybody says them. Then one day
you find the one person who you are honestly
put here to be with and you realize that
now when you say those things,
you really mean them."[1]

—*Billy Bob Thornton, on his marriage to
actress Angelina Jolie*

*D*eceptive unions are sown from the beginning of the romance. To make your relationship more satisfying, we must return to that first chance meeting in the smoky bar, the first held gaze across the wedding reception ball, the first words spoken as you met at the door to go out on your blind date. We must look at the key patterns that were established early in a relationship to understand why it has not met its potential to personally fulfill both partners.

Mirage men begin their relationships with the creation of artificial intimacy. This is established in an encounter between a man and a woman by emphasizing physical involvement with no regard to true compatibility. Usually one will hear this phenomenon described as "love at first sight," but it also occurs in initially unattached individuals who are eventually hormone-driven into each other's arms.

Artificial intimacy actually involves both a physical attraction to each other and a type of *approval seeking* we refer to as Phase 1. This involves a submersion of the man's true self so he can easily conform to the woman's tastes and thus heighten the sense of commonality between them. Any superficial congruencies in beliefs, interests, and goals will be seized upon to justify the tremendous sexual attraction between the couple. These similarities become a reason to believe in the future of the relationship. You hear it in the smitten suitor who exclaims, "I've just met the most wonderful woman. She jogs and laughs at all of my jokes!" He won't be able to rationally communicate why this lady is so different from the rest. It is this overwhelming desire that drives the relationship into the realm of deception.

Woody Allen's Academy Award–winning film *Annie Hall* features a scene that serves as an excellent example of this first stage of the syndrome. In this scene Woody Allen's deceptive character, Alvy Singer, is attempting to convince his new acquaintance (Diane Keaton as Annie Hall) that they share a serious interest in photography. Humorously, in this film Allen shows in captions what both people are really thinking as they speak:

❖

Allen: So, did you do those photographs in there, or what?

Keaton: Yeah, yeah, I sort of dabble around, you know? *(I dabble? Listen to me! What a jerk.)*

Allen: They're, they're wonderful! You know, they have a quality. *(You are a great-looking girl!)*

Keaton: Well, I would like to take a serious photography course. *(He probably thinks I'm a yo-yo.)*

Allen: Photography is interesting because, you know, it's a new art form and a set of aesthetic criteria have not emerged yet. *(I wonder what she looks like naked?)*

Keaton: Aesthetic criteria? You mean whether it's a good photo or not? *(I'm not smart enough for him. Hang in there!)*

Allen: The medium enters in as a condition of the art form itself *(I don't know what I'm saying . . . she senses I'm shallow.)*

Keaton: Well . . . well, to me, I mean, it's, it's, and it's all instinctive. You know, I try to get a sense of it and not think about it so much. *(God, I hope he doesn't turn out to be a shmuck like the others!)*

Allen: Still . . . still, you need a set of aesthetic guidelines to put it in a social perspective, I think. *(I sound like FM radio . . . relax!)*[2]

As we see in this example, the mirage man uses approval seeking to conjure up an atmosphere of immediate intimacy. While Woody Allen's character, Alvy Singer, couldn't care less about photography, he scrambles to establish commonality with Diane Keaton's character, Annie Hall. In the artificial intimacy stage, the woman is amazed that the mirage man shares so many of her likes, dislikes, and passions. We get to see in the movie *Annie Hall* that the mirage man is merely overwhelmed with sexual attraction.

The mirage man will not rely on just conversation to entice the woman into a romance with him. He has learned from his peers and the media what women enjoy in courtship, and he will use it as a weapon. Late-summer dinners at sunset-dappled cafés, slow dances in darkened dance clubs, moonlight walks along the beach, bittersweet love ballads and poetry, invocations of fate bringing you together, and pledges of eternal love will all be implemented in a rapid fashion to obtain the woman's trust and secure as much physical contact as she will allow.

Once the mirage man has found a woman who doesn't reject his initial flirtatious overtures, the mirage man will direct his efforts to maneuver the fledgling romance into the physical realm. The love he professes in his two-hour long phone conversations and ten-page love letters is mere sexual longing and infatuation with the superficial knowledge of the woman. Artificial intimacy created through approval seeking will mislead both lovers into thinking they have found "the one," and the religious among them will maintain it is "God's will."

In our sentimental society, this has become the common pathway to the altar. Contemplate the testimony of Steve, a thirty-four-year-old businessman, who met his future wife Steph at a Valentine's Day party. Steve stayed up talking to Steph until dawn and became engaged three days after. After marrying little more than a month later, on the day before Easter, the new groom proclaimed, "Once I knew that this was the right person, that we were meant to be, there was no point in waiting."[3]

Three days from meeting to engagement? Marriage in six weeks? It sounds rash, youthful, and even stupid. But responsible, mature, intelligent men are initiating such relationships every day across America.

Consider multimillionaire Mort Zuckerman. Several years ago, this brilliant, suave, sixty-something confidant of presidents, among the most coveted of Sunday morning political talk show guests, married Marla Prather, forty, the distinguished head of the Department of Twentieth Century Art at the National Gallery of Art. Said Prather, "We had a very short courtship, and then boom, we're pregnant. We're still getting to know each other and learning to be parents."[4]

Even the finest, most mature products of our top academic institutions are committing to virtual strangers now, getting to know their mate later. Predictably, this mirage marriage between academic giants was weak. In this case, Zuckerman and Prather chose to end their mismatch a few years later.

We laugh when uneducated younger couples are practicing foolish courtship and marriage, like heavy-metal rock star Tommy Lee and former *Baywatch* actress Pamela Anderson, who married after a four-day courtship.[5] When the marriage ended bitterly with charges of infidelity and physical abuse, we knowingly nodded.[6] What we have refused to acknowledge is that the same behavior is practiced by the leaders of our country in every walk of life. While we cluck our tongues at Tommy Lee, we ignore the fact that there are older and allegedly wiser couples like the Zuckermans behaving in similar fashion, with similar results.

Regardless of education, profession, and social status, we are seeing men use deception to deny women a mutually fulfilling, companionate relationship. These same men will maintain that they are merely seeking an intimate relation-ship. What could be wrong with that? The problem is these men have mistaken true intimacy for physical contact and sexual intimacy.

Let's define terms so that there can be no mistaking the damage mirage men do to themselves and others in seeking relationships with women. True intimacy, as defined by psy-chologist Harriet Lerner of the Menninger Clinic, is "a rela-tionship where one can be one's self and provide space for someone else to do the same, where we deepen and refine the truths we tell each other, where we hear each other and talk to each other about sensitive information."[7]

In contrast to an intimate relationship, a mirage man decides *not* to be himself. He sees that the woman is at least marginally interested in him or has use of him. She may not necessarily be attracted to him personally but may need some male to fill a temporary position in her life, such as a dance partner; an escort to the theater, ballet, or a formal affair; or as a confidant or a candidate to father her children before her biological clock strikes midnight.

Like a good door-to-door salesman, the mirage man takes advantage of this "foot in the door" of the woman's life. He uses approval seeking to win her over. He does his best from the onset to present himself as he thinks the woman wants him to be (Prince Charming, a bad boy, an intellectual equal, a likable rogue). Whether or not the woman practices honesty in the relationship, the mirage man is committed to living a lie. He rationalizes his behavior as the necessary cost of gaining sweet affection.

It is thus impossible to have a mutually fulfilling companionate relationship of true intimacy when the romance is predicated on artificial intimacy. Yet millions of American men are practicing this on their unsuspecting girlfriends and wives every day. Its prevalence demonstrates that somewhere along the way, American men forgot the meaning of courtship. Instead, these mirage men treat courtship and mating like the stereotypical male method of shopping for clothes on a weekend morning—they find the first thing that fits and rush home to watch the ball game. Only later will they notice if the colors clash.

Courtship was designed to ascertain the correct partner for each individual. There was supposed to be some discernment involved, some weeding out of inappropriate candidates, as in a job search. Today, American men are often entertaining any personality and temperament as a potential mate, from moody graphic artist to poised family practice physician, from shy librarian to boisterous improvisational comic. Yet our supposedly less enlightened forefathers and foremothers knew that the fitting of square pegs into round holes led to relationship disaster.

Although the mirage man is not discerning, we are not saying that he will take any woman to be his mate. Many men have a standard based on beauty and the basic acceptable rules of behavior of their culture from which they decide who to pursue and who to leave alone. Any woman at or above their standard is considered a potential partner. Instead of using the dating process to sort through these potential mates to determine compatibility and shared interests, the mirage man looks to any woman who meets his basic standard and will accept her as wife or living together material.

Mirage men are making life-determining decisions based on a look, a laugh, or the sparkle in a woman's eyes. There is no difference in result than the arranged marriages of *Fiddler on the Roof* or *Anna Karenina*, matchmaking and "store-bought" spouses of a supposedly less-enlightened era. Consider the following excerpt from an essay written by a man of forty-five and a woman of thirty-three, engaged two months after meeting:

We met,

We danced,

We fell in love . . .

He makes me feel like a love song . . . [8]

This is the groom's second marriage and the bride's third. With such discernment, is it any wonder?

Another couple recounted their courtship in this manner: by the second date the man "knew" they would marry. He asked her to marry him on the third date, and she declined, saying they didn't know each other well enough. Undeterred, he asked her to marry him on the fourth date. Somehow, one date later, she was persuaded that she knew him well enough and accepted his proposal. But the groom noted, "We look back and realize how little you know about the person, and how much intuition plays its role."[9]

Once the mirage man has found a datable woman who accepts his advances, he will begin his romantic offensive to secure his prize. He will devote all his time and energy to achieving his goal of eternal physical satisfaction and companionship. Whether this person is compatible with his personality or shares any of his true interests is irrelevant to him at this point. They may not even share a common language, but his goal in life is to convince her that they are in love.

In a fraction of marriages, the mirage man cheats the hangman and through dumb luck matches with someone compatible with his personality, with similar interests, values, and goals. Reading about those who did find a modicum of happiness despite deceitful means is like reading about state lottery winners. More likely are the marriages that fall back on the patriarchal marriage notion of separate spheres for each mate working toward the goal of perpetuation of the family by procreation. Otherwise there is no reason for marriages between strangers based on deception to last longer than the thrill of the honeymoon.

Today's ominous marriage and divorce statistics bear witness to the fact that mirage relationships are a long shot at best. Logic is definitely in short supply in the intoxicating high of artificial intimacy. Neither man nor woman is immune to the unbelievable optimism that everything will work out for the couple "in love."

Grammy and Academy Award–winning singer Carly Simon described the rapture of artificial intimacy when she met her first husband, singer James Taylor, in the early 1970s. Said Carly, "We were together a week and we decided to have two kids. One would be named Sally and the other Ben."[10] One week together and the couple had already selected names for their children? This is not unusual in the artificial intimacy stage. The euphoric feeling that washes over the couple destroys all judgment. Doubts about compatibility issues and differences in tastes, values, and goals eventually lead to estrangement, divorce, and the never-ending search for soul mates.

The Tiger Woods Syndrome is based on this false optimism of romance: love is a fairy tale, and once Prince Charming finds his princess, they will live happily ever after. Unfortunately, finding someone to accept your romantic offerings does not result in mutual personal fulfillment. Writer Morris Street succinctly summed up this familiar pattern of artificial intimacy when he wrote of his own experience: "Man meets woman, man woos woman, rockets go off, romance blooms, then the bubble bursts and reality sets in. Unfortunately, I've been involved in this pattern too often."[11]

Mirage men like Street have been practicing this pattern of courtship and marriage and are continually shocked at the ultimate negative result. Caught in a great collective insanity, they limp away from their last romantic disaster, exclaiming they are swearing off the women they blame for their troubles. Then a day, a month, or a year later, they use the same failed technique of romance in their next amorous adventure.

Actor Kelsey Grammer, star of the hit television shows *Cheers* and *Frasier*, is a typical mirage man. On the *Late Show with David Letterman*, he described how he had been twice married for nine months. On this talk show he revealed how he met his fiancée of the moment in a bar two days after filing for divorce from his second wife. He described staring at her from across the bar for an hour before a "voice" told him to go over and talk to her. Like Morris Street's experience, the rockets went off again for Kelsey. What he didn't know at the time of this television interview was that reality would soon set in before the wedding day, and this engagement would be broken. Kelsey has since married another woman. Apparently the "voice" was wrong!

Kelsey Grammer was inadvertently presenting a classic example of using artificial intimacy to begin another romance. Raw physical attraction across a smoky barroom and the belief in a preordained outcome do not equal a happy companionate relationship. Like most mirage men, Kelsey's unhappy history of cohabitation/marriage and estrangement/divorce seems to follow a familiar pattern of predictable heartbreak. Yet to this mirage man, the tragic results seem unconnected to the obvious cause.

In this chapter we have examined the first stage of the Tiger Woods Syndrome. The man will say what the woman wants to hear in order to achieve his ultimate goal of physical intimacy. However, the words spoken at this preliminary stage become less important as the aura of closeness envelopes the couple. The relationship is predicated on pure physical attraction. Many one-night stands end at this stage. If the relationship is going to progress from this initial deceitful beginning to something more permanent, the mirage man is going to have to start *living* the false image he has sold so successfully. Admitting deception is no longer an option. He will need to move into a new phase if he wants the deceptive romance to last.

6

I JUST WANT TO BE YOUR EVERYTHING: STAGE 2— *APPROVAL SEEKING*

"Good-bye, old friend.
This is the end of the man I used to be,
'Cause there's been a strange and
welcome change in me.
For once in my life I have
someone who needs me.
Someone I've needed so long."

—From the song *"For Once in My Life"*

*O*nce the mirage man has plunged into a new romance based on artificial intimacy, the second phase comes into play. The mirage man's focus turns from establishing the beachhead of the relationship through artificial intimacy to nurturing and strengthening the incipient union. The deceptive man knows that many a fledgling romance has faded after a promising first meeting. He will successfully continue the momentum of the deceptive romance by meeting the woman's many needs and desires so she will continue to mistakenly believe that he is the man of her dreams. For at least the short term, he will ignore his own needs, feelings, and desires in his attempt to constantly please his mate. This is the second stage of the syndrome, known as approval seeking.

The June 27, 1994, *Late Show with David Letterman* interview with movie star Alec Baldwin illustrated the deceptive behavior of mirage men in the approval-seeking stage. David

Letterman prompted Alec to share about his courtship of the beautiful Academy Award–winning actress Kim Basinger. Alec immediately launched into a vivid description of the character he played as a dating man known as "Mr. Sensitive." Alec realized Kim possessed strong vegan beliefs so to create an instant commonality he proclaimed that he was a vegan himself. He waved off the waiter who was going to bring him his usual osso buco and they shared the vegetable plate. Kim was convinced he was sincere and the relationship flourished. The immediate effect was sentencing him to a diet of what he called "spicy dust": beans and rice and covert trips to In-N-Out Burger. Alec described the long term effect: ". . . to impersonate Mr. Sensitive and then to live it, for the relationship to succeed, and now that I'm married, and to carry on the charade of Mr. Sensitive in an ongoing way, is exhausting."[1]

Alec Baldwin achieved his short-term goal of snaring one of the most beautiful women in the world. Unfortunately, he couldn't keep up his Mr. Sensitive routine. His true self, initially hidden under the seat like an In-N-Out Burger wrapper, came to dominate their marriage. As Kim Basinger's father recounted, Kim repeatedly warned Alec, "You've got to overcome this anger, or I can't live with you." Attempts at counseling were fruitless, as Mr. Sensitive had achieved his short-term goal and no longer had the desire to please Kim by consistently attending marriage and family therapy appointments. Further, he could no longer pretend to adapt to her desire to live in Los Angeles instead of his beloved Long Island. With the mask of Mr. Sensitive discarded, the true Alec was too much for Kim, and she separated from Alec after seven years of marriage.[2]

We see examples of this deceitful, short-lived Mr. Sensitive not only with famous actors but with everyday people all around us. Consider a Notre Dame High School football player who was nicknamed "The Alien" because of his eccentricities. Once he met his current girlfriend, a Notre Dame High cheerleader, he appeared to change. He reported that suddenly, "I'm normal. My girlfriend has a good effect on me." But his coach, Kevin Rooney, knows better, adding, "He's far from normal. He's 'The Alien.'"[3]

Could it be that this young man changes whenever he is around his girlfriend? After all, his coach still maintains he's the same outlandish kid out on the gridiron and in the locker room. This is a typical example of the second phase of the mirage man. The changes in the mirage man in this second stage can be subtle or dramatic. Whether he changes his car radio presets from heavy metal rock to hip-hop, begins attending and participating in his girlfriend's church, develops a craving for vegetarian food she adores, or spends all his free time with her family on weekends, it all points to this second stage: approval seeking.

Actor Charlie Sheen is a vivid example of the approval-seeking male. He announced that he was divorcing his wife of six months because he had married the wrong person, really wasn't ready to get hitched anyway, and, in retrospect, should have taken more time to get to know his wife (supermodel Donna Peele) whom he'd wed after a six-week courtship. Shortly before his marriage, Sheen testified in the trial of Hollywood madam Heidi Fleiss, admitting under oath to ordering Fleiss's prostitutes at least twenty-seven times at a cost of more than $50,000.

Like most mirage men, Charlie Sheen eventually found the Mr. Sensitive persona he had adopted to win a supermodel to be overwhelming. He said, "I couldn't breathe. I like breathing too much. I had to come up for air."[4] Given Charlie's lifetime history of hedonism, one can imagine the horror his new wife experienced when Charlie decided to "come up for air" and be his true self. If only he had given her the chance to choose or reject the real Charlie Sheen before their whirlwind courtship and wedding. But that is what mirage men do in the second stage of the Tiger Woods Syndrome: they deceive their girlfriends for the "good" of the relationship.

The mirage man may not always purpose in his heart to intentionally deceive his new lover. He may even delude himself into thinking that he likes all the things his girlfriend likes. But by seeking her approval at the loss of his true self, he slowly and steadily misleads her into confirming her hopes that she has found her Prince Charming at last.

Consider the woman's perspective during the approval-seeking stage. *Sex and the City's* Kim Cattrall costarred in the CBS TV movie *Every Woman's Dream*, a real-life account of a mirage man who lived a double life with two separate wives who were both oblivious to their shared husband's twin deceptions. Regarding the theme of the film of romantic deceit, Kim commented, "Making the film, I wondered how women could have been so deceived—but then I realized the smartest of us can be so stupid. I started to look at my own life and some of my bad past relationships, how little I really knew about them."[5]

Under the current system of dating and mating, we are all capable of ending up in a committed relationship with a stranger. Kim Cattrall is a perfect example. She was so close to the truth. She could easily see the folly of the cuckolded woman in her television movie. Her character showed the importance of learning about a man before committing to him romantically. Yet at the time of this movie, Kim was involved in a mirage relationship, preparing to marry a fellow actor (*Murder One*'s Daniel Benzali) she had only known for eleven months. She rationalized that it was okay for her to rush into this marriage because "I know absolutely everything about him . . . Daniel and my relationship [*sic*] is based on truth and honesty." Well, maybe not everything. This engagement blew up like a rocket on the launching pad just short of liftoff, but a year later the irrepressible Kim was featured in the news, planning a wedding with another man she has known for *four months*. She says, "We've been together ever since [meeting], and are now headed toward marriage."[6] This marriage ended abruptly after three years. Like many American women, Kim was caught in the insane romantic loop of participating in the same deceptive courtship behavior of artificial intimacy and approval seeking with mirage men over and over, wondering why she wasn't getting better results.

Writer Eric Adler describes the subtle process by which romantic true believers like Kim are misled as "little lies, blatant fabrications, deliberate omissions, secrets kept about actions or thoughts: all are part of the panoply of falsities that can creep into relationships and even reside there permanently."[7] In the approval-seeking stage, the man uses these "little lies" to deceive the woman into thinking she has found a lover who will listen to her, share her unique interests and life goals, and love her with all of her faults.

Phase 2 of approval seeking is more significant than the Phase 1 approval-seeking that we discussed in Chapter 6. This type of approval seeking is much more serious and intense. There is tremendous pressure on the man at this stage of the relationship to keep it going strong. He is like the fisherman in Ernest Hemingway's *The Old Man and the Sea*. The more effort he expends trying to land his romantic "catch," the less likely he is to cut his line and move on, even though the mounting evidence indicates he is wasting his time with an incompatible mate. He is going to make this relationship work out like he wants—no matter what the cost. Control is a major issue for mirage men, even though they appear to be giving control of the relationship over to the woman at this stage.

In addition, the religious mirage man has the added burden of proving after the fact that the physical attraction and any sexual activity that occurred during the artificial intimacy stage was justified because they share so much in common in the mental and spiritual dimensions. It cannot be countenanced by such "moral" mirage men that they had engaged in casual sexual behavior with a virtual stranger. It is in this second stage that the religious mirage men are driven to conjure up the illusion that this romance is with their unique soul mate, predestined by a higher authority.

In this phase, the mirage relationship moves past mere superficial commonalities and raw physical attraction and is now based on the lie that the man shares so much of his new girlfriend's background, interests, tastes, and goals. Unlike the artificial intimacy stage, the man is now firmly committed to a lifestyle of pleasing his new love every day. He has to put in time and energy to prove in a hundred little ways that he is her Prince Charming. The couple develops a history at this stage. Shared books, concert series, dances, weddings, birthdays, and holidays spent with each other's families harden the cement of the relationship.

In the approval-seeking stage it becomes impossible for the mirage man to backtrack and admit his true feelings, tastes, and goals. Once he has made his commitment to the physically based relationship, he is stuck with trying to fit his personality and tastes around hers.

Todd, an eager twenty-four-year-old glove salesman, knew he couldn't tell his girlfriend that he was pretending to like the honey-baked ham that was regularly served Sundays at her parents' house. He continued to act as if it were as much a treat for him as it was to her family. He believed that even sharing his true conflicting opinion on something that trivial might lead her back to the multitude of other little lies he had spun since the romance began. Todd knew that if she ever discovered how he despised her family as much as the ham, he would be exposed as a fraud and the romance would come to a screeching halt. He learned to live in a world of deceit, often referred to by this mirage man as "white lies."

Much as he may protest, there is no denying the mirage man is a fraud at this point in the relationship. His girlfriend doesn't realize it, but the mirage man is using a skill that is gender-specific to men: disconnection. According to Terrence Real, a senior faculty member of the Family Institute of Cambridge and co-director of the Harvard University Gender Research Project, men are forced to disconnect from their feelings early on, first from their feelings for their mother "for fear of sissifying them," all in the name of being a man.[8] Once in school, boys learn by their junior high years that even when they have a legitimate reason to cry due to insult or injury, they are to deny their feelings or be ridiculed by their fellow males as a "crybaby." Boys come to realize that feelings are the enemy of manliness and must be denied continually. By adolescence boys have learned that the art of being a man is to put up with anything to achieve a given goal.[9]

Sadly, the cost of suppressing emotions is high for men. As therapist and author Marvin Allen notes, "It's like going to the dentist to have your tooth filled. In order to stop the pain of one tooth, the dentist has to numb the whole side of the jaw."[10] Thus, young men have a reduced capacity for a wide range of emotion that women take for granted.

Mirage men bring this time-tested method of denying their true feelings to attain their prize. They see courtship and marriage as another time to hide their emotions, just as they did in the playground kickball game, the paper chase in the classroom, and in competing on the social ladder for friendship. A mirage man will listen to a woman go on and on about herself and her problems for hours on end if he believes a kiss and more wait for him on the other side of the conversation. Chameleon-like, he will adopt her values, interests, and goals if he thinks it will result in short-term physical satisfaction.

A good example of this behavior is found in former

Partridge Family television star turned talk show host/disc jockey Danny Bonaduce. He boasts that he has been married to his born-again Christian wife, Gretchen, "for five years, and we've known each other for five years and seven hours." According to Danny, "It didn't bother me that I married a stranger in order to get sex from a woman who didn't want to have sex until she was married." Danny used artificial intimacy to plunge into the marriage. He used approval seeking to maintain it, ceding all control of the relationship to his wife. As he phrased it, "I'm not captain of the ship at home. I'm barely first mate."[11]

Danny Bonaduce isn't the only mirage man attracted to religious women. A recent report on devout Christians married to nonbelievers noted that the vast majority of these "unequally yoked" Christians are women. True to the syndrome, a significant number of these women reported marrying "men who pretended to be Christians during the courtship only to reveal their religious indifference after the wedding."[12] Their approval seeking was successful in getting them to the altar. Living the 100 percent Christian life after the wedding was another story, as their shocked and disappointed Christian wives were to discover.

Ironically, the approval-seeking technique that the mirage

man uses to win his woman ultimately prevents him from having an emotionally rewarding relationship with her. According to psychologist Harriet Lerner, deception in a relationship creates distance between the partners and "erodes connections and blocks authentic engagement and trust, and strips the couple of spontaneity and vitality and keeps them operating on a higher level of anxiety."[13] Thus, in the mirage man's determined quest for an intimate relationship with a woman, the deceptive means result in a physically intimate relationship without the capacity for true emotional intimacy.

Whether he is a misogynist mirage man or a compliant mirage man, both kinds of mirage men use the approval-seeking stage to perpetuate their fledgling relationships. The misogynist mirage man will appear to have few, if any, boundaries. His perfect behavior will prompt his girlfriend to wonder aloud to others if he ever gets angry about anything. Sadly, this good Dr. Jekyll behavior is merely an act that will end abruptly later in the fifth stage of the mirage relationship (resigned compliance, which we'll discuss in Chapter 9). In this terminal stage of the relationship, the real Mr. Hyde emerges. His anger issues will then dominate the relationship, and he will not have any desire to please his mate by seeking professional help to correct it.

The compliant mirage man will be indistinguishable from the misogynist at this approval-seeking stage. He will be completely devoted to the task of pleasing his woman and losing himself in her opinions, tastes, and goals. However, in the fifth stage of the syndrome, the woman may discover his slavish devotion is not genuine, and she will lose all respect for the wimp who will grovel in the gutter for a relationship.

At this point in the growing mirage relationship, the man becomes a prisoner of his own device. He could opt for honesty and begin to express his true self to the woman, at the risk of losing the union. He will usually choose the winning formula of minimizing his own tastes to avoid conflict and perpetuate his image as Prince Charming to his Cinderella.

In Tiger's case, he could have told Elin during their courtship that he didn't wish to be committed to one woman because he enjoyed promiscuous sex. But that would have ended the relationship, so he pretended to be the kind of husband she always wanted. The sad results now involve two other human beings who will always wonder what happened between Mom and Dad.

The mirage man's greatest fear at this early stage of the relationship is that the truth about his real self will leak out to the woman, and the romance will disappear in a puff of smoke. These anxieties are usually unfounded. Telltale clues of his deception, like Alec Baldwin's In-N-Out Burger wrappers lying on the floor of his car, will usually be ignored. Why? The nectar of physical intimacy, effort expended, and the seductive romantic fantasies of the woman discourage painstaking inspection of the aberrant behavior by the misleading male. Yet, if she did do the necessary detective work, expose him for the cad he is, and end the relationship at this approval-seeking stage, there would be a minimal amount of permanent emotional damage and time wasted.

We are nearing the crucial turning point. If the courtship strengthens in this phase, serious and long-lasting commitments will be made based on false pretenses. The relationship will be caught up in a powerful swell toward permanence. In Chapter 7, we will see that the cost of deception increases exponentially as the relationship moves into commitment/ abandonment, the third stage of the Tiger Woods Syndrome.

7

WHEN A MAN LOVES A WOMAN: STAGE 3— *COMMITMENT/ABANDONMENT*

The best mirror is an old friend.

—George Herbert (1593–1633)

*O**nce the mirage man has** established a relation-ship based on artificial intimacy and strengthened the illusion of love through approval seeking, he is faced with one more challenge to his sham romance. Although the sky looks bluer and each snowflake shines like a diamond to the smitten man, reality soon intrudes on his dreamland of infatuation. He is forced to choose between the old realistic life he has left behind and the new fantasy lifestyle he has adopted to please his new partner. This is stage three: commitment/abandonment.

Inevitably, the real world and the deceptive male's fantasy world collide when he introduces his old male friends to his new lover. These friends represent the mirage man's real self, established over years of good times and bad. These primary relationships are carved out over the years to meet the man's varied tastes and needs, ranging from emotional intimacy to competition. These friends exact a "buffering effect" on the man. They keep him from wide behavioral swings, just as a buffer solution resists drastic changes in the body's acid level. Changes in mannerisms, speech, style, and personality are instantly challenged with hoots of derision, sarcasm, or a raised eyebrow from the knowing chums who exert a scouring peer pressure that corrects unreasonable behavior. This correcting mechanism will come into action when the mirage man brings his phony relationship into the real world of his friends.

Sometimes there are some embarrassing incidents that prompt the woman to confront the mirage man about his "awful friends" who seem so different from the caring and polite man she has been dating. She will stand in astonishment as one of the mirage man's friends relates an ancient story of crude or lewd adventures. She will kick her Prince Charming under the table while another old friend shares an off-color or politically incorrect joke. Strongly held opinions expressed in the safety of trusted friends appear like ghosts, coming back to haunt the man. Worst of all, the deceptive man's spin on his life will be open to challenge by his friends and acquaintances. Instead of a happy homecoming, the mirage man will suddenly realize how Neanderthal his gang of acquaintances has become.

Many deceptive men avoid this pitfall by dating women outside their friends' social circle. Then they can live a dual life: their Prince Charming persona with their girlfriend and their normal persona with their friends and family. Unfortunately, even the mirage man who dates outside his friends' social circle begins to feel pressure as the relationship moves from artificial intimacy to approval seeking. As his time commitment to his girlfriend increases, the deceptive man must cut back on his time spent with his friends. If he works full-time and has other involvement in the community, he will soon discover he has no time left for his friends without cutting back on the time spent on his blooming romance. Something has to give.

The deceptive male will now feel forced to choose between his lover and his old life. He will feel sadness and regret as he realizes he must abandon relationships he once felt were so precious to his day-to-day existence. But he has already sold his soul to start the relationship. The romance has priority over everything else in his life. In addition, the dissonance these old friends could create if they intruded on his new life is one more good reason to act. He will feel compelled to abandon his old life completely if he is to continue his romance.

Often the rapidly progressing relationship itself forces the issue. The mirage man may be forced to make a sudden choice between the new girlfriend and his old life, symbolized by his friends. Tomas, a twenty-eight-year-old entertainment executive, was faced with such a dilemma when his girlfriend of eight months pressured him to let her move in with him in the apartment he shared with his childhood friend. When the friend objected, Tomas angrily moved out and ended the lifelong friendship.

Such is the way with the third stage. Bridges are burned that can never be rebuilt. Indeed, this is the critical point of no return in the development of the syndrome. The mirage man has distorted his life to please his mate, but there is still time to renounce his deception before his actions begin to have permanent consequences. Sadly, this is a rare occurrence. Very few men have the guts to admit they are behaving in a reprehensible manner.

It did occur to Scott, a twenty-one-year-old Moorpark Junior College student. He had just met an attractive sorority girl at his brother's fraternity exchange with the Zeta Tau Alpha sorority. To establish immediate intimacy, Scott pretended he was a member of a University of Southern California (USC) fraternity. The combination of superficial commonality and sexual attraction had its desired effect of artificial intimacy that evening. But after several dates, Scott was saddled with guilt and remorse. The relationship was moving into the second stage: approval seeking. He wanted the relationship to continue. But sooner or later he would have to introduce her to his friends and family (Stage 3). How could he explain then that he was a "lowly" junior college student, not the dashing Scott from USC? The relationship ended when he courageously admitted his deception, shattering the growing trust between the couple.

The mirage man will not tolerate his friends' and family's warning that his new lover is not compatible with him in the least. Never mind that they know his tastes as well as he does in his more sober moments. The mirage man will ignore their advice even if the friends and family can clearly show that the new mate is dangerous, destructive, and even criminal. Jamaal, a thirty-two-year-old high school basketball coach, gave up his beloved Boston Celtics when he moved in with a new lover with a substance-abuse problem. When he placed his roomful of Celtics regalia in storage, Jamaal was symbolically placing his true self in storage to perpetuate a deceptive romance. Jamaal's friends and family all opposed the romance with a shiftless party animal who detested sports.

Jamaal cut off all ties to his friends and close-knit family because he didn't want their uniformly negative views to influence him or convince the woman to leave this good person alone. He adapted to her world as much as he could in his search to find someone to love.

This shunning of friends is illustrated in the classic Percy Sledge song "When a Man Loves a Woman":

> *When a man loves a woman*
> *Can't keep his mind on nothin' else,*
> *He'll trade the world for the good thing he's found.*
> *Yeah, if she's bad he can't see it.*
> *She can do no wrong.*
> *Turn his back on his best friend if he put her down . . .*

Here the mirage man, like Jamaal, is described in detail. He has distorted his personality to please his lover. He will no longer value the buffering effect of his friends as they pose a threat to the phony image he has presented to his new love interest. Any reasonable criticism of his new love will be used as a pretext for abandoning relationships that took a lifetime to develop. If his new lover suffers from addictions or mental illness, he will deny it. All that matters to him is perpetuating the relationship based on physical attraction. Abandoning friends and family is an easy decision for most mirage men.

Some mirage men never choose between their old life and a new relationship, because the old life is *another* relationship! A Los Angeles private investigator describes this especially virulent form of deceptive male who has *hidden* his old life for a relationship:

❖

"Out here on the West Coast, the usual line is that they're a professional athlete or an actor. But one guy told a woman he was a dentist, but didn't have a phone number. In the end he had a wife but no dentist's license . . . You'd be amazed at how so many women have dated guys for months and only have a pager number for him. They don't know where he lives, and most of the time it's because he's got something to hide. This year's most intriguing case would have to be an 80-year-old guy with a wife in her 70s who was busy seeing several girlfriends in their 20s. The guy is truly amazing."[1]

Tiger Woods never gave up his old life for Elin. He became an expert at living the dual life and had more than a dozen girlfriends on the side and used prostitutes as well. Beloved CBS newsman Charles Kuralt was another one of these amazing mirage men who lived a dual life. Until the venerable reporter died in 1998, his legions of fans and his dutiful wife and children had no idea he had a thirty-year "on the road" relationship with Patricia Shannon. After he died, Shannon asserted that Kuralt had promised her a Montana ranch, and she wanted to claim it.[2]

Peter Contos is another example of an extremely busy mirage man who lived a dual life. Contos lived with his wife and her parents in Stoneham, Massachusetts, while maintaining another girlfriend who bore him two sons only fifteen miles away in nearby Lowell, Massachusetts. Contos convinced both women that his frequent absences were due to U.S. Air Force duties, when in fact he had resigned from the air force and actually worked some security jobs and served in the National Guard. His trademark mirage man technique was to call and say, "I can't give you the number where I am, but I'll call you right back." It bought him years of living a dual life.[3] In fact, his secret life may never have come to light had it not been for the murder of his mistress and children (he was tried and convicted of the murders in 1999).

Serial cheaters Tiger Woods and Peter Contos symbolize the fraudulent nature of all mirage men in this third stage of the syndrome. If the mirage man does not admit his deception to his girlfriend at this point, he will abandon his old life for his deceitful romance. He will adopt the phony approval-seeking role as his true self. With the abandonment of his friends, he will soon forget who he really is. Without the buffering effect of his past, he is free to portray himself as Mr. Sensitive to his poor, misled mate with no fear of contradiction.

Author and therapist Marvin Allen describes the result of a generation of deceptive men choosing women over their old friends: "Few men have lasting friendships with other men. It is common for a man to have only one intimate relationship, the one with his female partner, and to keep other people at arm's length. He has business contacts and acquaintances, but few close, continuing friendships."[4]

It wasn't always like this, but modern American men tend to be alienated from other men and have an unrealistic dependence on their wives and live-ins to supply them with all their companionship needs. In contrast, in addition to their husbands, women usually have "eye-to-eye" friends with whom they can share openly, which helps them meet their emotional needs. Today's men tend to be "Lone Rangers" who look solely to their wives or live-ins for personal support. When these mirage men do spend time with other men, the time is spent with "side-to-side" friends in activities like sports, which keeps things detached and safe.[5]

The mirage man will rationalize that he doesn't need his friends and will concentrate on his lover to provide him with all his needs. Although popular music and film will encourage him that this is true, it is impossible for one woman to meet these demands. Sociologist and author Dr. Robert Ackerman describes the irreplaceable importance of strong male relationships in a man's life: "If men ever talk about their problems, it is usually with women. However, we only share with women what we think a man should share with women. Whether we are aware of it or not, there is an unspoken line about what we talk about with women that few men will cross. We don't talk about men's issues with women. We don't talk about how it feels to be a man. We can talk a little about our pain or express some emotions, but it is not the same in sharing it all with another man."[6]

Men need men in their lives, as well as their spouses. By

abandoning his friends, the deceptive male will put undue and unreasonable expectations on his unsuspecting mate to meet all his relational needs.

The mirage man, by consciously leaving his friends, destroys relationships that took years or even decades to mature to a satisfying level of intimacy. He will find it frustratingly difficult to create new friendships that will have the depth of his old confidants. He can construct a picket fence of acquaintances at his work, sports leagues, service clubs, and church, but he will find himself hemmed in by strangers. He will always have to hold his true personality back in fear that his deception to his woman will be discovered and publicized.

Especially disastrous will be attempts at friendship with other deceptive males, as real sharing is impossible with other men who are also using phony personalities. Likewise, male bonding movements like the Christian-based Promise Keepers will be exercises in futility for a man who has a secret identity. He may feel emotional catharsis in singing stirring religious hymns with 100,000 other men in a stadium, but no healing of his dishonest soul will take place. He has too much to lose.

Often a woman will sense the ache in the deceptive man's

soul at the long-term loss of his friends. She may encourage him to try to revive these lost bonds to his past months or years later, but by then it is usually too late. The old life has been shunned. His friends know they are not worthy of inclusion in his new life. The broken trust is difficult to mend over a once-a-year ball game, a high school reunion, or a special boys' night out. The deceptive man has committed himself to playing a role far from his true self. With his good friends gone, there is no one he can relate to. His future is that of a very lonely man. He will be surrounded by strangers who think they are his friends and a wife who can't understand why he is so resentful and emotionally frozen.

The mirage man avoids dealing with the consequences of his deception. He is consumed with living in the moment. He will leave his true self to conform to his mate with little regret. Now he approaches the payoff to his deception: the honeymoon. In Chapter 8, we will see why millions of American men become chameleons for love.

8

WE'RE IN HEAVEN: STAGE 4— *THE HONEYMOON*

"Sometimes you have to get to know someone really well to realize you're really strangers."

—*Mary Tyler Moore*

I n an earlier America, men did not cut themselves off from their friends and relations once they found a new romance. The concept of courtship was originally designed to link honest men and women of compatible temperaments and shared interests and weed out mismatches. There was no need for guile, for withholding the reality of each other until some far-off day after irreversible commitment was made. It seems hard to believe, but once upon a time, Americans did not fear the truth.

In the 1800s, the prospective bride was integrated into the man's life. If she could not abide his friends and relations, it was considered proof of incompatibility, and the courtship would end. That was the point of courtship. Instead of dating like an ostrich with one's head in the sand, the fact that two people might not be compatible for a lifetime commitment was faced with eyes wide open. Early Americans knew that a man's friends were a mirror of his true self.

This common-sense approach to courtship and marriage was lost in the early twentieth-century American zeal to be modern. Now the typical American male denies the truth that he and his prospective mate might just be mismatched, like Tiger committing to a Swedish au pair. This rush to commitment reaches its zenith in the fourth stage known as the honeymoon. At this time the relationship takes on a tone of life-altering permanence.

In Chapter 7, we explored the events leading up to a monumental decision for the mirage man: being forced to choose between his old life and his new lover. He may make this decision with agonizing consideration or flippantly within seconds. One thing he knows for sure is that his future plans have hit a defining fork in the road.

In Stage 4, the man is still practicing approval seeking, conforming in every way to her vision of the perfect man, but he is slowly finding this chameleon act is creating tremendous stress in his once-serene life. He is trying to please his girlfriend by devoting all his free time and energy to her, but somewhere in the back of his mind is the nagging memory of his old life, symbolized by his friends and family. They understand that the man has found "true love," but they also expect him to spend some time with them like before. With his disappearance stretching from weeks to months, the pressure builds on the mirage man to integrate his girlfriend into his established life.

In the era of healthy dating, this task of integrating his mate into his existing life would already have occurred during the initial courtship, but in the modern era, the mirage man is not portraying his true self to the woman. Whether he is a compliant mirage man like Tiger Woods or a misogynist mirage man, at this stage he is facing the moment of truth in cementing the future of this relationship. He may be the compliant mirage man who loves his woman and completely adapts to her life willingly. On the other hand, he may be a misogynist mirage man who pretends to be Prince Charming but is ticking like a time bomb with hidden hatred of all womanhood, including his new lover. Regardless, he is threatened by the growing possibility that this new lover will discover the truth about him. He fears that once she gets to know his uncouth friends and dysfunctional family, she will see that his courtship persona of Prince Charming is a fraud. Instead of coming clean, he will do anything to avoid her discovering the truth and ending the relationship.

This abandonment of his friends is reinforced by the media. Men have been taught for generations that one must choose between his love and his friends. Film critic Joan Mellen notes, "When men in American movies are heterosexual and share their lives with a woman, they are generally deprived or incapable of friendships with men. From [Marlon] Brando in *On the Waterfront* to [Humphrey] Bogart in *To Have and Have Not, The Big Sleep,* and *The African Queen,* the model of masculinity in films is presented with an implicit choice: if he would link up with a woman, he has disqualified himself from enjoying male friendships."[1]

The big lie promulgated by Hollywood is that a heterosexual relationship will provide all your relational needs. This leads millions of men to believe that they don't need the friendships of other men, as they are just poor substitutes until that truly all-satisfying relationship with the love of their lives comes along. Supported by the media and driven by desire, a decision will be made at this critical stage: the unsatisfying past or the incredibly happy future? Given the mirage man's infatuated state of mind, logic is lightly considered in his final judgment. Seeing the Holy Grail of eternal companionship and sexual ecstasy so tantalizingly near, most mirage men choose the sham romance.

Once he has made his choice of the relationship, the mirage man intentionally or passively abandons his old life and completely devotes himself to his new lover. The couple will be completely physically intimate, even if they have delayed such gratification for moral/religious reasons. They will rationalize that it is okay to have sex now since they are so committed to each other. If the couple is young and seeks mere cohabitation, they will move in together. But if the couple is in their mid-twenties or older, and marriage has become the ultimate goal, short- or long-term engagement plans will surface now.

In Stage 4, the couple experiences the emotional euphoria popularly known as the honeymoon, with weeks or even months of bliss. Bestselling author Dr. Harville Hendrix describes this brief interlude as a time for couples when "fears are held at bay . . . and romantic love is going to heal them and make them whole."[2] To the lovers, the relationship will always be one of true, unconditional love. It is the mountain-top experience all mirage men have dreamed of since junior high school days. For the deceived women, it is their Cinderella fantasies come true.

Tony, a once-divorced thirty-five-year-old truck driver, enjoyed such a peak experience with a striking thirty-three-year-old woman he had known for a little over three months. For this couple in love, every day was one of joy spent with each other. In each other's presence, they couldn't keep from holding and kissing one another. All day long, Tony would receive text messages from his beloved from her workplace telling him that she loved him and would see him that night. Drunk on the honeymoon experience, he ignored the warnings of family and friends, quit his job, sold his house, and moved to Memphis to begin a new life together. Tragically, he returned two years later—unemployed, broke, and bitterly divorced.

Tony's sad refrain was, "I wish I had gotten to know her better first." After the fact, one can plainly see that the Tiger Woods Syndrome has terrible consequences, but those on the peak slope of the honeymoon experience ignore the warnings of a coming storm.

The rapture of the honeymoon reassures the mirage man that he has truly made the right decision in choosing romance over his old life. Although he has conjured up this relationship through the dishonest tools of artificial intimacy and approval seeking, to him, the ends more than justify the means. "My friends are just jealous!" he rationalizes to himself. The mirage man will comfort himself with the knowledge that his friends and family will never experience the oneness that he is presently enjoying with his mate. He wants to believe they would do the same thing if they were in his shoes.

The mirage man's friends realize they are being abandoned during this honeymoon stage. Usually there is not some grand announcement or royal snubbing, but a slow and steady withdrawal by the mirage man from all emotional involvement with his friends and relations. At first it will not be noticed, as the mirage man has been scarce since his new romance began. But there is a distancing that occurs in this stage that is distinct. Eye contact will be averted and once in-depth conversations will abruptly remain at the superficial level. The mirage man will give narrative on how great his romance is going, but his emotional range will be even more limited than before.

A friend will inquire about getting together for a regular activity and the mirage man will defer to his girlfriend for an answer. He may still give lip service to getting together but will become extremely elusive if definite dates and times are proposed. His voice has the new sound of moving on to a new stage of life with his new "best friend," his girlfriend. There is no more room for male friends in his new life of romance. The hard truth hiding behind his forced smile is that the only real use he has for his old friends and relations is as groomsmen and an audience for a future wedding.

The abandoned friends and relatives react in three ways to their abandonment: suffer silently, express their hurt through guerilla warfare of well-timed sarcasm, or go ballistic. Matt, a twenty-two-year-old college student, faced one such nuclear reaction after he stood up his two best friends for set plans when his fiancée became available at the last minute. Once an inseparable threesome in their fraternity, the friendship began to wither on the vine once Matt began a mirage romance with a cheerleader. When Matt didn't even have the nerve to call his waiting friends to break their plans, they took matters into their own hands. The next day Matt discovered his car completely covered in trash. It was a symbolic reminder of what this mirage man had done to his two primary male relationships. Typically, Matt refused to take responsibility for his poor treatment of his friends. He retaliated in kind to their cars, escalating the war between them. Characteristic of the honeymoon stage, many relational bridges were broken.

Regardless of his friends' and family's reaction to their abandonment, the mirage man moves on with his life. He is focused only on the product of his trickery, his burning-hot romance. He hopes love will take care of every worry. Matt summed up the unrealistic view of the mirage man on his wedding day. Caught up in the thrill of the honeymoon stage, he exclaimed, "Now all my troubles are over!" This compliant mirage man didn't foresee a loveless ten-year marriage that would end in adultery and divorce.

Thanks to a deceptive courtship, the mirage man has misled the woman into believing she has found Mr. Right. The relationship is now predicated on his continued portrayal of this fictional character. More pressure will build for the mirage man to conform his will to his partner's to continue the fantasy of romantic love. Through the loss of all moorings to his true self, the mirage man will find himself committed to the full-time job of deceiving his new mate.

In the short term, the mirage man shrugs off the loss of his friends and relations as the cheap cost of sweet, physical intimacy. If the relationship ended at the honeymoon stage due to unforeseen tragedy, like the star-crossed lovers in the movie *Titanic*, there would be nothing but great memories to comfort an aging spinster. But in the real world, as the deceptive union wears on, the mirage man will begin to loathe the person he has become. Then the thrilling honeymoon stage will fade away to the harsh reality of incompatibility, leading to the fifth and final stage: resigned compliance. The Dan Fogelberg song "Make Love Stay" reflects the fear the mirage man feels at this moment of greatest happiness:

Now that we know
The fire can burn bright or merely smolder,
How can we keep it from dying away?
Moments fleet, taste so sweet within the rapture
When precious flesh is greedily consumed
But mystery is a thing not easily captured
And once deceased not easily exhumed.

This is the fear of anyone who has engineered a relationship based on artificial intimacy and approval seeking: how do we keep the honeymoon high from ending? Unfortunately, it would be easier to walk on water than keep the relationship from hitting its inevitable bottom. Sexual attraction and memories of passionate nights definitely have the power to keep couples bonded to each other for a while. The reality that the partners have little in common besides their passion will become very significant in Chapter 9, where we will look at what happens to the mirage couple when the sexual "mystery" inevitably dies. The union can't stay new and fresh forever. The passion cools and compatibility issues take the place of rapture, which ultimately occurs as a predictable result of basing the relationship on deceit.

9

AFTER THE THRILL IS GONE: STAGE 5— *RESIGNED COMPLIANCE*

"The good Lord set definite
limits on man's wisdom, but set no limits
on his stupidity—and that's not fair!"

—*Konrad Adenauer, German statesman (1876–1967)*

*H*ollywood lost a favorite fun couple when super-
star actors Bruce Willis and Demi Moore
announced they were ending their more than ten-year marriage. The couple divorced after two years of sporadic media
speculation that things had soured for the once-passionate
lovers. But is it any wonder? Bruce and Demi had known
each other for three months before marrying in a nearly mil-
lion-dollar wedding.[1] Like other mirage couples before them,
they believed that sexual attraction and a white wedding day
could overcome incompatibility and diverse needs, feelings,
and goals. Eleven years later the Willises stand as living testimony to the folly of the syndrome.

Tiger Woods did the Willises one better, spending almost
$2 million for a sunset wedding on the island of Barbados—
yet the result was the same. Bruce and Demi and Tiger and
Elin were fooled just like millions of other romantic true
believers in the power of the honeymoon. But in reality, the

honeymoon is a mirage, a fantasy based on the basic dishonesty of men begun early in the dating/courtship process. The honeymoon's brief interlude of total isolation from the harsh truth of the relationship is the emotional peak of the syndrome. Many couples like the Willises and Woods look back months or years later wondering what went wrong, and more pragmatically, how to get it back. But despite well-intentioned groups like Marriage Encounters, the problems of two mismatched people bound together cannot be seriously dealt with in a weekend seminar. Reality will not allow the couple to retreat into yesterday's deception once again.

The honeymoon begins to fade as the mirage man begins to sense the terrible cost of achieving his goal of eternal companionship and physical satisfaction. He has reached the final stage: resigned compliance.

In resigned compliance, the mirage man takes off his rose-colored glasses and surveys the increasingly hopeless scene he has created. He has previously denied his legitimate needs, feelings, and dreams to please his mate and achieve eternal companionship and physical satisfaction. Initially this was not burdensome, but eventually the strain of keeping up the charade that his lover's tastes are his own takes its toll on the deceptive man.

In resigned compliance we see the weakness inherent in mirage men. It is a short-term solution for a long-term relationship. In the movies, Robert Redford, George Clooney, or Cary Grant only had to be charming for two hours. But the mirage man is expected to live his phony persona for the rest of his life. Not surprising, the mirage man slowly wears down over time. He becomes an actor who must portray Mr. Sensitive twenty-four hours a day, with no flubbed lines or missed cues. He is not allowed to take off his costume, wash off his greasepaint, and relax with a smoke in the comfort of his dressing room. He has a fully committed partner waiting in the wings who believes with all her heart in the character he is depicting. Every scene requires his presence as Prince Charming. He soon finds himself trapped in his deceptive role.

The mirage man's seamless performance will inevitable begin to slip. His mate will begin to see disturbing glimpses of another, more unpleasant man as the physical intensity of the honeymoon stage begins to wane. For the mirage man, the pain of living with someone of few common interests, differing worldview, and clashing temperaments will become acute. Physical intimacy will lose its painkilling potency as the relational differences come creeping out from beyond the shadows into the light of day.

The relationship will now decline in three steps: realization, disillusionment, and crisis. These steps will have similarities and differences for the misogynist and the compliant mirage man. Let's look at each of the three steps in detail:

Step 1: Realization

Whether he is a misogynist mirage man or a compliant mirage man, the relationship is now in decline. A misogynist mirage man who has pretended to be Prince Charming to gain the relationship is now close to exploding in his pent-up hatred of all womanhood, focused specifically at his new mate. On the other hand, a compliant mirage man who loves his woman has willingly adapted his whole life to please her. Both the misogynist and the compliant mirage man realize at this stage that they have committed themselves to a life of obligation. It was easy for them to put up with a three-hour opera and a carriage ride in the park when the evening culminated in fresh, sweet, physical intimacy, but now the healing balm of love is fading. It becomes harder and harder for both the misogynist and compliant mirage man to stifle their tastes and feelings when they receive a diminishing reward. The inherent conflicts in the relationship become harder for the mirage man to ignore as the thrill of the physical aspect of the relationship wanes. Soon the irritation and pain become greater than the prize.

Both the misogynist and compliant mirage man are challenged to create a long-term strategy that allows them to function in the relationship without destroying it. They must accept as a premise that one must give up any notion of returning to his true self. Their goal is to continue in the physical part of the mirage relationship. To do this the mirage man will carefully negotiate areas and times when he can express small fragments of his real self without threatening the union. He will create events that he knows his mate enjoys around events he really likes.

For instance, if his wife detests sports but favors social events, he will suggest attendance at New Year's Day gatherings and Super Bowl parties, or join a golf and tennis country club so he gets his sports fix while she is entertained. If she is worried about her figure, he will sign them both up for a fitness club membership so he gets to play basketball, volleyball, and racquetball while she does Pilates and swims. If he actually gets her to go to a sporting event, it is sandwiched between a lavish pregame picnic and an expensive postgame dinner with another couple. These win-win events work well for a couple with little in common.

Both the misogynist and the compliant mirage men will also try to do the things they really like around the margins of their mate's plans for the day. For instance, if his wife or live-in is a late sleeper, a mirage man will get up at 5:30 AM on a Saturday morning to play golf. If the round of golf takes longer than the expected four hours and fifteen minutes, the mirage man will walk off the course on the sixteenth hole rather than risk being late for his woman's planned daily schedule. He certainly can't tell her to wait, as he presented himself as a man who didn't care about sports that much at the beginning of the romance. Her plans have always taken priority over his secret desires for the weekends. He knows he must live out this deceptive role for the happy illusion of love to continue.

The day-to-day grind of living a role that isn't genuine leaves both the misogynist and the compliant mirage man feeling weary, oppressed, and resentful. They will be careful not to alienate their wives or live-ins through a tidal wave of pent-up rage. The mirage man will instead learn to express these feelings in sarcasm, bickering, and simmering, never-resolved arguments about non-relational subjects like the family pets, and home-improvement projects. He thinks this is a safe way to blow off steam without revealing the real reason for such a well of unending anger. The wife or live-in is none the wiser about her mate's deception, and the mirage man releases his resentment at his mate and himself in short increments. A mirage relationship can function for years and even decades using this technique of venting anger. Eventually, the resentment leads to the next step in resigned compliance: disillusionment.

Step 2: Disillusionment

In this step the mirage man becomes exasperated with his mate as the potency of the physical aspect of the relationship wanes and the clashing of different temperaments and lack of common interests and goals takes center stage. This is the unavoidable result of both the compliant and misogynist mirage man's tactic of keeping his true feelings to himself. The once-passionate relationship between the mirage man and his woman begins a long, slow slide toward estrangement. In this phase the process of falling out of love occurs. Florida State University psychology professor Dan Boroto attributes the death of love as a "direct result of undisclosed communication."[2] Withholding information worked well for the mirage man during the artificial intimacy and approval seeking stages, but you can't cheat the hangman. The same deceptive technique that was used to perfection to win the romance is now the agent of destruction in the resigned compliance stage.

The wife or lover of the compliant or misogynist mirage man experiences a slow, steady disillusionment about her Prince Charming in this second step of resigned compliance. Her once-affectionate swain is now distant. The constant stream of flowers and love letters reduces to an irregular trickle, then finally dries up completely. Her eyes may be as blue as ever, but she doesn't hear him talk rapturously about them anymore. Sure, they are doing most of the things she envisioned most couples do, but there is something amiss.

Now there is a startling new downward spiral in the relationship. Both the compliant and misogynist mirage man ooze resentment in their actions and obsequious manner in complying with the most mundane requests they used to jump to eagerly. For example, some of the kindest and friendliest mirage men will suddenly snap into a trance of irritating and bizarre behavior when the wife or live-in interrupts him just to ask a question. These disillusioned mirage men will agree to take the family on a Sunday drive into the country in the sport utility vehicle instead of watching the football game, but they will tool along ten miles below the speed limit just to signal their anger at having to do one more thing they hate doing. The wife cannot understand it. "Didn't he say he was a devoted family man when we were dating?" she will muse. The innocent bystanders, the children, will never understand why Daddy is so touchy. The wife or live-in of a mirage man begins to lose faith in the relationship as the Prince Charming morphs into an unpredictable grouch.

Compliant and misogynist mirage men are poor communicators with their wives because they fear the consequences if they show their true selves. These men believe it is less threatening to their marriage to hide behind a wall of silence and enjoy a low level of happiness than reveal their real feelings and risk losing the cohabitation or marriage immediately. In Tiger Woods's case, imagine what would have happened if he had casually mentioned his propensity for porn stars? No wonder writer Lesley Dorman observed in *Redbook* magazine that "What are you thinking?" are the four most terrifying words a woman can say to a man.[3]

Truly, this is the tragedy of the syndrome. The compliant or misogynist mirage man has sold himself to his woman as her Prince Charming. When the woman buys into the persona the man portrays, she is defrauded into purchasing a myth. Her experience is similar to that of someone who buys a house based on a picture in the real estate section of the local newspaper. When she shows up in a moving van with all her belongings ready to move in after escrow closes, she discovers that the house is a facade like those used in B-grade westerns. There is no depth or substance to the person she has committed to, merely an attractive exterior. As Elin Nordegren discovered, all the wealth and fame in the world can't substitute for a real relationship.

Consider the legendary singer/actor/comedian Dean Martin. He certainly was an icon of masculine cool to generations of young males growing up from the 1950s to the 1960s. Dean was a member of the 1960s Rat Pack (which also included Frank Sinatra, Sammy Davis Jr., Peter Lawford, and Joey Bishop) starring with the rest of the members in the original Oceans Eleven, and was the host of a top-rated variety show on television featuring the beautiful "Golddiggers" dance troupe. Fans were assured "Dino" was a wonder with the opposite sex. But his second wife, Jeanne Martin, revealed in a 1978 interview that Dean Martin used the same failed technique as other mirage men with the same terrible results, quipping, "When I met Dean Martin, it was love at first sight . . . I married him knowing nothing about him. I divorced him twenty-three years later, and I still know nothing about him."[4]

Mirage men do not know what women want. They think they have fulfilled their part of the bargain. They have sold out their true selves to gain the relationship. They resent the fact that their women want more. Women want to get to know their men. Mirage men like Tiger Woods know that is the one thing they cannot allow, or the relationship is over. Therapist and author Marvin Allen echoes the cries of millions of mirage men who are backed into a corner by their wives or live-ins who demand more than complete obedience.

> . . . the real surprise for me in my marriage was that my
> wife wanted more from me than money and sex. It wasn't
> enough for her that I was working as hard as I could six-
> teen hours a day. It wasn't enough for her that I was an
> indefatigable lover. It wasn't enough for her that I had
> given up seeing my buddies, chasing women, playing
> sports and going fishing. She wanted something more
> from me, something that I found impossible to give: inti-
> macy. I was keeping such a tight rein on my feelings that
> there was no way I could let her get close to me.[5]

Here Marvin Allen freely admits going through the first four stages; artificial intimacy, approval seeking, and choosing the relationship over the old life symbolized by his friends were no problem. But now the honeymoon is fading for this driven mirage man, and he is resistant when his wife naturally tries to develop the union into greater intimacy. Like all mirage men, he feels he must remain alienated from his real self to perpetuate the romance born of dishonesty.

Over the long haul, this ends up destroying the marriage or cohabitation. Sonya Rhodes, a marriage and family psychotherapist and author of *Second Honeymoon: A Pioneering Guide to Reviving the Midlife Crisis*, observed the damaging effect a poor relationship has on the sexual aspect of marriage. Through her years of clinical therapy, she has observed that women tend to see sex as a natural result of a healthy relationship, while men consider sexual relations unconnected to the interpersonal aspect of the marriage or cohabitation. When a marriage is ailing, the sexual relations tend to be withheld by the woman, while a married man "wants to have sex even when the relationship is under stress." Dr. Rhodes urges women to address the issues of conflict in a marriage openly so that women will be "less likely to use sex as a weapon."[6]

Because both compliant and misogynist mirage men have learned to deny and hide their true feelings about the mirage relationship, they are not likely to transform into emotionally available communicators at their well-meaning wife or girl-friend's urging to address the conflicts threatening the marriage or cohabitation. The mirage man is afraid his wife or live-in will think he is a "scum of the earth" if he vocalizes his underlying issues about their union.[7] He wants to have sex even when the relationship is under stress because he has *always* had sex while under the psychic stress of knowing he has been deceiving his partner since the mirage relationship began. He is merely acting in the committed relationship as the same goal-oriented, deceptive man he was in the early dating relationship.

The compliant or misogynist mirage man remains emotionally withdrawn from his increasingly miserable wife or live-in to preserve the relationship, lest he be found to be a fraud. He will ironically discover that the main reason for creating the deceptive relationship, namely sex, will diminish as the wife or live-in's opinion of their relationship wanes. The deceptive man will find his moments of physical intimacy declining with his partner's declining opinion of the emotional intimacy of the union. She will find her efforts at communication cut short by her emotionally frozen and resentful mate. In a snowball effect, the woman will tend to communicate her growing displeasure about the relationship by becoming increasingly withdrawn physically.

To both the compliant and misogynist mirage man, this is fighting unfair. No matter how poor the emotional relations are on a daily basis, he feels his primary source of physical affection should continue to flow unabated. Bestselling author Dr. John Gray observes that the resentment is temporarily washed away for men when they enjoy regular sexual relations in a committed relationship.[8] Thus, the well of anger dwelling deep within the mirage man increases as his physical relationship with his partner declines. As therapist and author Marvin Allen observes, the relationship shifts from one of romance to one of conflict.[9]

As painfully obvious as this is to women, men are blind to the reason why the physical relations in a mirage relationship decline. They have no idea why their fed-up mates withdraw physically from them. Marriage researcher Pepper Schwartz terms this resulting scenario as the most common type of sexless marriage, where "there's a lot of anger and two people who simply don't know how to change their behavior.[10] However, it is mirage men who do not even think there is any behavior to change. They actually feel victimized by their partners when they are denied privileges. These men gather in locker rooms and bowling alleys, card rooms and beer halls to commiserate with one another, rationalizing that this is the way all marriages and cohabitations end up. They feel no personal responsibility for their present predicament. All they know is "they aren't getting any!"

The result of this second step in resigned compliance is a bumper crop of bitter, self-absorbed men who are oblivious to their disintegrating marriages and miserable cohabitations. Disillusionment now leads to the third step of resigned compliance: crisis.

Step 3: Crisis

In the crisis step of resigned compliance, both partners end up miserable. Both the mirage man and his wife or lover realize that the reasons they had fallen in love were myths. The woman discovers that her dream man is in fact a mirage—someone who never really existed except in her mind. She kept expecting her husband or boyfriend to behave like his Mr. Sensitive persona of courtship in their committed relationship, but she finally realizes it was all an act. She will be wounded by the hard truth that her lover grovels and pleases her for physical affection, while not even liking her as a person or, in Tiger Woods's infamous text message, feel a connection to her. Meanwhile, her mirage man will be despondent with the hard reality that he will not enjoy the sweet physical libation of the honeymoon stage. Both partners sense the hopelessness of their shared situation.

Terror is a shared emotion between the mirage man and his deceived wife or live-in within the crisis phase of resigned compliance. They must both deny the terrifying truth that their union is built on a foundation of deceit. The hardest hit is the woman. She knows she has been deceived by her mirage man—that Prince Charming was a frog after all. No matter what she does from this point on, it will be very difficult for her to recover from this devastating deception by her trusted man. Psychologist John Northman has found that the victims of betrayal, through hard work, can build a level of trust back up, but the initial betrayal will never be forgotten.[11] For people who live in a small town, or someone who is high-profile like Tiger Woods, the betrayal can be so profound that only by moving away can one avoid the constant reminders of it.

In Chinese philosophy, crisis is both a time of danger and

opportunity. In the mirage relationship, this crisis phase is a time when the harsh truth must be faced. The question is, will this truth be buried in denial or will the opportunity be seized to save the committed union? This can actually be a time for healing as well as destruction. There are five possible outcomes for the compliant and misogynist mirage man and his deceived mate in the crisis step of resigned compliance: hitting bottom, returning to insanity, calling a truce, ending it, or having what we call special deviant mirage relationships, all of which we'll look at in detail now.

Hitting Bottom

The couple may hit bottom, meaning they realize their union is in serious trouble beyond their ability to mend it on their own. This is the best of all possible outcomes. The compliant or misogynist mirage man will begin to own up to his role in the destructive relationship. Despite the bleak outlook, both partners commit to the idea of staying together and want to exhaust every avenue to save the marriage or romance. They will seek outside intervention, including marriage counseling, psychological services, 12-step groups for codependency and individual addictions harming the partners, and other resources. For instance, Tiger Woods would need to confront a possible sexual addiction before the marriage could be saved. (This will be addressed in detail in Part Two: Recovery and the Mirage Man.)

Return to Insanity

The second outcome is for the compliant or misogynist mirage man to step back from the cliff and take into account the cost of ending the relationship. Fearing the consequences of divorce, other legal and financial costs, and trauma to his children, many mirage men will fashion an apology to their wife or live-in and return to pretending to be Prince Charming. This occurs after many of those weekend marriage encounter–type therapies and Promise Keeper rallies.

In this outcome the blame for the crisis in the relationship is placed squarely on the mirage man. But the solution is not a search for the true man and a new relationship based on honesty, but instead a return to the deceptive ways of courtship before the honeymoon ended. Thus, artificial intimacy and approval seeking are seen as positive values that can save the union instead of the very actions that led to the current pathological marriage or cohabitation.

In this return to insanity outcome, the mirage man redoubles his efforts to conform himself to his mate once again. The mask of Mr. Sensitive is placed back on his face. His wife or live-in will accept the repentant mirage man back into her good graces, but things will never be the same as before, as she is now armed with the fact that his compliance is all an act. If he begins to rebel later, she is quick to bring him into line as the phony he truly is.

Return to insanity is a Band-Aid approach to relational cancer, as it does not deal with the fact that the relationship is built on deceit. Many a "good" marriage that once tottered on the brink of destruction was saved by the mirage man repenting at the crisis stage and resuming his phony act as Mr. Sensitive.

Truce

The third outcome during the crisis phase is the common, cowardly reaction of many people to the harsh reality facing them: the mirage man and his wife or live-in deny it and go on with their relationship with the unspoken agreement that neither will mention the awful truth again. Both the mirage man and his mate know that things are not right. That is the terrible secret they must both carry around with them for the rest of the relationship. But anyone can see that they have transformed from attentive lovebirds to two prickly porcupines bristling with resentment. Watching them force a kiss in public is a painful spectacle to behold.

Mirage men who react in this manner during the crisis phase will use a common defense mechanism of unhappily married men everywhere who have seen their dreams of eternal companionship and physical satisfaction dashed on the rocks of reality: they will withdraw to cope with the estranged relationship with their wives. Withdrawal is the socially acceptable way for both the compliant and misogynist mirage man to paper over the chasm of differences between him and his mate. The actual way each man will withdraw varies.[12] Overeating, serial adultery, workaholism, religious addiction, sports and card-playing addiction, excessive television watching or reading, pornography, gambling, controlling and fixing others, and fixation on their children and grandchildren's lives are but a few of the more than 180 addiction behaviors identified by Dr. Gerald May.[13] They may also rely on chemical painkillers such as alcohol, tobacco, prescription pharmaceuticals, and street drugs and narcotics. The goal of all these behaviors is to protect the mirage man from the reality of his self-created hell on earth.

Ending It

Realizing the hopelessness of the situation, many couples separate and file for divorce. This may be done immediately, or it may be a delayed reaction after years of existing in the return to insanity or truce phases of the crisis step of resigned compliance.

Usually the mirage men will stay in the disintegrating relationship until they can trade up for a new partner or wait until the kids grow up. Once the beauty fades and the romance is but a dim memory, an increasing number of mirage men know what to do with the stranger they committed to: they dump her for a younger woman.

This linking of older married men with young ingénues has certainly become a phenomenon of our American culture. The movie *The First Wives Club* connected with women who had been betrayed by mirage men, who had deceived them into long-term relationships, only to be abandoned years later for younger women.

Such was the case with Georgia Waller, the wife of romantic icon Robert James Waller. After thirty-six years of marriage to the author of *The Bridges of Madison County*, Mrs. Waller filed for divorce. Despite his claims that Mrs.

Waller was his inspiration for the heroine of the bestselling book and hit movie, Robert abandoned his wife for a fling with the younger forewoman of their Texas ranch.[14]

This is the sad future for many women who have bound themselves to mirage men. These deceived women will spend the best years of their lives with men frozen in an emotional hibernation from them. The mirage man they commit to may eventually physically abandon them for other women if the opportunity presents itself. But even if the mirage man stays faithful to the marriage, they practice mental cruelty on their wives through their intentional and willful neglect of them.

This withdrawal eventually leads many long-suffering spouses to take the initiative and file for divorce after years of trying to make the marriage work. The sad reality is that today in America, women are filing for divorce twice as often as men, and the usual reason is that they have been emotionally abandoned.[15]

The purpose of this book is to spare women across America from the poisonous fruit of compliant and misogynist mirage men. These charlatans of love never did care much about what their women said from the moment they met, as long as it was positive toward the mirage men themselves and furthered their ultimate goals in the relationship. Mirage men will appear to attentively listen for hours to their women to gain a relationship during the artificial-intimacy and approval-seeking stages. But once the physical libation of the union decreases after the honeymoon stage, mirage men will see little reason to devote themselves to the emotional needs of the strangers they have committed to. The wife of a mirage man will end up emotionally abandoned whether or not she is physically abandoned.

Deviant Mirage Relationships

A fifth, more troubling outcome of the crisis phase of resigned compliance involves one of the partners accommodating the disturbing behavior of the other. In other words, due to psychological defects in the partners, the mirage relationship appears to thrive in the crisis stage for years or even decades. There are two distinct types of this strange behavior: the masochistic compliant man and the controlling woman and the misogynist man and the compliant woman. First we will look at the masochistic compliant man and the controlling woman, a derivative of the compliant mirage man relationship.

The Masochistic Compliant Man and Controlling Woman

The masochistic mirage man displays the character defect of enjoying the mental pain of a poor relationship. He actually enjoys getting treated like the worthless person he knows he is and searches the world for the woman that will make him feel that way. Thus, he is attracted to women who display the character defect of control.

During courtship the masochistic male will accede to all of the woman's wishes through the honeymoon stage, but during the resigned compliance stage, the woman will begin to notice that while her man still agrees with the letter of the law of family life, his heart is no longer in his work. He will kindle a simmering resentment from living with an incompatible mate, but never openly rebel against the controlling woman. He will attempt to find opportunities to covertly do the things that he really likes. He won't let on that he doesn't share his mate's beliefs, goals, and dreams. Eventually, she will realize that her Prince Charming has no genuine core beliefs besides pleasing her. She will lose respect for the spineless man who stands for nothing. Then the magic of the marriage will be over.

In this case, it is the controlling woman and not the

masochistic mirage man who realizes the marriage is in the crisis phase. To continue in the union from this crisis point on, she will learn to seek her pleasure in things outside of the relationship. Peer relations, career, children and grandchildren, the arts, extramarital affairs, community service, and sports are but a few of the ways she will distract herself from the depressing fact that she was misled into a commitment with a wimp who fears her rising voice. She will decrease physical affection approaching zero as a reflection of her poor opinion of the relationship.

The masochistic mirage man will hold on to the relationship at any cost. He will accept the limited physical relations in the union as the cost of living his whole life with her. He will be forced to accommodate his increasingly resentful mate and end up a caricature of the henpecked man, constantly striving to please but never satisfying his emotionally distant wife. Due to his character defect of enjoying abuse, this will drive him all the more to preserve the marriage.

The controlling woman has a right to be angry at her masochistic mirage man. She will remind him of that every day they are together. But the compliant mirage man in this situation never gives up on the marriage. He is determined to give 99 percent to the 1 percent his withdrawing mate has decided to give the relationship. He believes he can make the union right through sheer willpower and complete obedience to her.

The relationship may remain in crisis for years with no resolution to the basic issue that the woman was deceived into a commitment. It is a continuing relationship, but it is as fragile as a balsa wood glider. It only continues to fly as long as the controlling woman is willing to put up with her love-servant. If some opportunity for substantial long-term romance presents itself, the controlling woman may opt for it as a ticket to escape a man she can dominate but not respect.

In this type of compliant mirage relationship, the masochistic mirage man will be the last one to know that the marriage is finished. He is aware that she may very well be cheating on him, but he will ignore the damning evidence all around him. He knows she wakes up each morning despising him for his treachery in establishing the romance, but he will be the one to put on the phony smile and pretend to his family and friends that everything is fine.

The Misogynist Man and the Compliant Woman

Another special case is the misogynist man and the compliant woman. A healthy woman would leave the relationship once the misogynist started to show his ugly true self.

But what of the women who are willing to put up with abuse from men?

For the misogynist mirage man, the resigned compliance stage quickly progresses past the initial phase of his realization that he has committed himself to a life of obligation with someone of few common interests and clashing temperaments. The pain of living with her increases as the potency of the physical aspect of the relationship decreases over time. All his anger at womanhood in general will be stored up and ready to unleash as the honeymoon begins to fade and sex no longer has its numbing effect on his damaged soul. He is fed up with pretending and kowtowing to her every whim. Now it is time for his real, woman-hating self to emerge.

The compliant woman who has been deceived by a misogynist mirage man has quite a surprise in store for her. As the relationship moves past the realization phase of resigned compliance, she is oblivious to anything being wrong. Suddenly, as the union declines into the disillusionment phase of resigned compliance, her dream guy begins to act completely out of character. She discovers to her horror that her Prince Charming is, in fact, a monster who continually plots against her plans for domestic harmony. All her fairy-tale dreams for happily ever after will fail.

A nationally syndicated column by psychologist Dr. James Dobson describes this form of misogynist mirage man in a question sent to him by a bewildered wife: "I'm certain that I'm losing my husband. He shows signs of boredom and total disinterest in me. He treats me rudely in public and is virtually silent at home, and of course, our sex life is nonexistent. I have begged and pleaded with him to love me, but I'm losing ground every day. What can I do to save my marriage?"[16] Dr. Dobson responds in the column with palliative care for treating the symptoms of a poor marriage. He advises the wife to back away and not pressure her "trapped" husband. But this does not deal with the fact that the relationship is based on deceit on the husband's part, and now the consequences of his deception are beginning to be reaped. As a mirage man, he used to pretend he was interested in her, and treated her politely in public. Now that the thrill of the honeymoon is gone, he treats his wife with abuse that he wouldn't heap on his hunting dog. This is the exaggerated reaction of a mirage man with serious women's issues.

On her solo album *Excerpts from a Love Circus*, Lisa Germano, the great violinist in John Mellencamp's band, captures the despair of women like her who repeatedly fall for misogynist mirage men who eventually turn abusive: "I've been that passive person who gave too much love, and it just hasn't worked . . . This record is really about three relationships I had that were all very similar. I was just repeating this pattern, and finally said to myself: 'Isn't it stupid to love someone who makes you feel irritated all the time?' Like, 'You have such bad breath and your breasts aren't nice,' you know? . . . The question I'm asking on this record is simply, 'Why do we choose people who make us feel bad?'"[17]

Lisa Germano and the hapless wife in Dr. Dobson's column capture the essence of the plight of a compliant woman bound to a misogynist mirage man in the misery phase of resigned compliance. These poor women do not know why the once-loving man they committed to is now so abusive. He has long since stopped trying to please his mate. In this phase he actively tries to humiliate and antagonize her. The mystified woman becomes demoralized when she realizes what he is really like. The issues that never seemed important during courtship now bring the misogynist to extreme anger. As the woman becomes convinced that she has bound herself to a monster, she realizes there is no longer a basis for a relationship, save the commitment they made and any children or worldly possessions they have accumulated as a couple together. The relationship then declines into the crisis phase, where several outcomes are possible.

First, the couple may realize that there is something here beyond basic incompatibility and, with the woman's urging, seek professional help for the misogynist man first and the marriage second. This character defect of the man looms large before anything can be done with the basic dishonest foundation of the marriage. But if the woman is willing to wait for the man to get psychological treatment for his hatred of women, then she might have the dedication to rebuild the union between two strangers from the foundation up (this topic will be further explored in Chapter 12).

Another outcome in the crisis phase of resigned compliance for the misogynist man and compliant woman may involve the woman's realization that this marriage or cohabitation cannot be saved due to the man's hatred and violent potential. Her actions may include gathering herself and any children and fleeing for both her emotional and physical safety. Only then will she file for separation and divorce. In this era of O. J. Simpson, it is obvious that misogynist men do follow through with their threats of violence, fueled by an untreated rage against womankind.

Another less-hopeful outcome is that the woman will try to preserve the relationship by compromising with some of her misogynist mirage man's less outrageous demands and accepting his new, emotionally cool self. Yet this appeasement only buys a temporary peace. The woman may react like the wife in Dr. Dobson's column who kept trying to behave in the same loving manner as she did in the early stages of their relationship. But her misogynist mirage man will rebuff her affectionate actions, since he has long since stopped playing his phony Mr. Sensitive role.

While the woman will do her best to keep the family unit functioning, the misogynist will continue expressing his true, angry self until all those around the couple—at work, church, and so on—will know they are desperately unhappy. All his long-hidden addictive and compulsive behaviors will come into full view of family, neighbors, and friends, yet it may take years or decades of thoughtlessness, cruelty, and even physical violence before the wife will quit putting up the brave front that her marriage is "happy." She will accept that her marriage, if not ideal, is "normal" and never seek help for all the abuse and shame she has to endure. Instead, she will transfer her passive role as a victim to her children, as a model for what they should expect in their future marriages.

In this chapter we have viewed the decline and fall of a marriage system built on a foundation of deceit. Despite the hopes of a white wedding, the mirage man and his spouse often end up completely miserable. Now that we see the cost of deception, let's explore how to heal yourself from a mirage relationship.

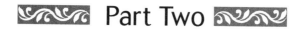 Part Two

RECOVERY AND THE MIRAGE MAN

10

HOW WOMEN CAN PREVENT MIRAGE RELATIONSHIPS

"New opinions are always suspected,
and usually opposed, without any other reason
but because they are not already common."

—*John Locke, English philosopher (1632-1704)*

Now that we know the five-stage pattern of the Tiger Woods Syndrome, how can women recognize these clever deceivers? The quiz in Chapter 2 is a good place to start. You should be able to use the quiz to see if prior relationships have been unhealthy, but how can you prevent the next relationship from being deceptive? And what of young women who are just entering the dating pool? How can they avoid these charlatans of love?

Sadly, because of the propaganda in film, television, videos, and music, women must assume that the average man has been brainwashed into accepting dishonest behavior as normal unless proven otherwise. With the widespread practice of hooking up or being joined at the hip, the average man assumes he will have superficial relationships based on physical attraction. Few men object to immediate gratification with no strings attached. This makes it extremely difficult for women who are seeking a romance and eventual marriage based on honesty and candor. Most twenty-first-century men simply aren't familiar with it.

Given this challenge, here are ten steps to having a mirage-free relationship:

1. **Insist on a healthy relationship from the beginning.** Men are most open to new suggestions for relating at the beginning. Later on they may fake cooperation but hold back to their old familiar ways that have served them so well.

2. **Develop your own interests and keep your boundaries.** It is crucial for you to develop your own interests and stay committed to them. Then you can meet men who share your passions. So many women have spent their lives doing things they hate to gain affection. All it does is feed resentment. Don't let that happen to you! While there is the chance that mirage men will worm their way into groups and pretend to like an activity, participating is a great way to increase your chances of meeting someone with whom you actually have something in common. The secret is to carefully study how your intended

partner behaves in the group or activity you attend. Is he there just to meet women, or does he have a commitment to the activity above and beyond the next relationship? Usually the scammers are blatantly obvious. It's sad to hear how many women say the last time they went dancing was when they met their present hubby. Don't be fooled by mere attendance.

3. **Determine if the man is honest.** When you first meet someone with whom you have something in common, follow several key guidelines. First, try to determine if he is being honest or is just telling you what he thinks you want to hear. If he is seeking your approval, you can assume he is a mirage man. Second, be aware if he seems too agreeable. That is a technique used by the mirage man to create an illusion of compatibility that will fade after the honeymoon stage. He should have some definite ideas that clash with your own, even if it is such trivial things as the time you meet, what restaurant you go to, and so on. If all his tastes are yours, he's conning you.

4. **Don't tell him your life story.** Mirage men base relationships on a phony notion of intimacy. These

dishonest men want to build an irresistible momentum that drives the romance into greater physical
intimacy by creating immediate mental intimacy.
Women can short-circuit this technique by fighting
the tendency to blurt out their life story on the first
few dates. The best thing you can do is respond to
questions but hold healthy boundaries on what a
virtual stranger should know about you. As the relationship progresses, there will be plenty of time later
to share confidences. This stops the undertow that
drives many deceptive-based romances to the altar.

5. **Risk confrontation.** While talking to your intended
partner, see if he is willing to risk confrontation. The
secret to this technique is to be aware of telling too
much too soon. The mirage man uses everything you
reveal to mimic your tastes and views. Instead of
blurting out all your tastes and views, let him go out
on a limb on a subject and then tell him you don't
agree with him. Watch his reaction. That will give
you more insight into what he would be like as a life
partner than anything else you could do. Does he
clam up? Does he fume? Does he seek compromise?

Does he accept the conflict, respect your views, and move on? This is what you want to determine before any emotional commitment is made. A healthy relationship deals with conflict.

6. **Watch how he reacts to taking things slow.** If you are playing the field, let him know that you are just interested in a friendship for the time being. Many mirage men will reveal themselves at this time. They are in a rush to close the deal like a real estate agent. You can spare yourself a lifetime with a jealous spouse by watching his reaction to the news that for the present time you are seeing other men and just want to be friends. In addition, that tells him he will have to take time to get to know you with no immediate physical payoff. That realization weeds out many mirage men and leaves those who are persistent and will make good partners.

7. **Meet the Fockers.** Once you begin dating, get to know his friends and family. They tell you what he is really like. Mirage men will fight this because they are chameleons who don't want to let you know their true selves. Consider any reluctance on his part to be

a red flag. If you have trouble getting along with his friends and family, consider it a blessing that you have found out before you are committed to spending all your weekends, leisure time, and vacations with them.

8. **Find his true self.** Encourage him to share more of his true self. Don't try to change him, because he will just go underground with his true self while appearing to change on the outside. If he sees he can trust you, he will be more willing to be honest with you and abandon mirage man behaviors. Think how much better it would have been if Elin could have found out that Tiger was addicted to sex *before* they were committed to each other. He might have been more willing to deal with it then, and if not, Elin could have spared herself from possibly being exposed to sexually transmitted diseases and being linked to Tiger through the children for the rest of her life.

9. **Avoid the honeymoon.** Fight the mirage man tendency that as your relationship deepens, you isolate yourself as a couple from the world. The honeymoon is a tool of the mirage man. Your relationship should

be just as enjoyable when you are in social situations. It should also be strong enough to sustain itself once the initial passion diminishes.

10. **Be ready for some shockers from the truly honest man.** Honesty can be a rude awakening when you have grown accustomed to the deceptive man's approval-seeking ways. Many women are genuinely shocked when their man unveils his true self, which may include a sex addiction. Many men are addicted to Internet pornography, and others like Tiger practice serial adultery or frequent prostitutes. Find out before you make irreversible commitments.

When the man does reveal his seamy side, don't just stand there dumbfounded. His disclosure requires reciprocal honesty on your part. Be ready to take positive steps and be supportive in helping him deal with the character defects and addictions he may reveal to you in confidence. For instance, if a mirage man reveals his sexual addiction to you, help him by avoiding situations that will cause him to struggle. Don't take it as a put down when he admits he is tempted in a specific moment. It may be as simple as avoiding steamy movies or his being able to tell you he needs to trade places with you at a restaurant because a skimpily-clad woman is sitting across the room in his line of sight. In our sex-drenched society this is a common occurrence.

Your own character defects and addictive behavior may also have to be dealt with after years of submersion. A tendency to enable deceptive pathological behavior may come to the surface. Seize this moment to improve yourself as he improves himself.

11

ROMANTIC RULES
FOR MEN

"Real relationships grow without
someone forcing them to grow
through artificial intimacy."

—*Dr. R. A. Richards II*

*N*ow *that we have explored* the scourge of the syndrome and defined the concept of a healthy relationship, how does the single man avoid the unhealthy tendencies in the rough-and-tumble world of dating? There is nothing worse than knowing that what you are doing is wrong yet not having the knowledge or skills to avoid repeating it. For that reason, this chapter deals with the changes in behavior needed after a man has changed his mind about practicing the deceitful modern method of dating. Men with a conscience will read this book and find themselves in a quandary: they can't go back to deceiving women, but how do they date in a healthy manner?

We've compiled the following rules for all age-groups, from the teen who is just entering the dating scene (or the parent advising him), to the widower who is seeking someone late in life, to everyone in between. These rules will help the novice of any age who wants to learn the right way to approach the opposite sex. In addition, these rules also apply to divorced men who have paid the steep price of broken relationships. The good news is that it is never too late to begin practicing these ten basic rules toward healthy dating and relating.

RULE NO. 1:
NO DATING UNTIL YOU CAN DRIVE

Pre-sixteen-year-old relationships beyond school-yard crushes can lead to traumatic sexual experiences: teen pregnancy, abortion, adoption, date rape, sexual abuse, fifty different sexually transmitted diseases, and, at best, mirage relationships. Common sense tells us: hang out in public with groups of guys and girls and keep sex hypothetical.

Most fifteen-year-old males feel enormous peer pressure to date as proof of their heterosexual masculinity. If they aren't seeing a girl, they feel tremendous shame. The inadequate fifteen-year-old boy will respond to these feelings with a variety of behaviors. They run the gamut from lying about imaginary lovers and exaggerated superficial friendships with the opposite sex to all kinds of reckless sexual behavior, including acquaintance rape and "parties" where more than one boy is sexually initiated by the same girl.

The media have lied to teens for forty years in shows like *The Wonder Years* and *Happy Days* by suggesting they are "missing out" if they aren't dating, when, in reality, early dating robs them of their adolescence. Millions of lives have been forever altered by this insane behavior that is condoned by many parents who can't or won't say no to their sons. What they have unwittingly done is put more pressure on their unprepared children to go out and perform. Parents: be the bad guys and allow your sons a scapegoat they can blame so they don't have to live up to society's destructive new standard of virility.

RULE NO. 2:
DEVELOP YOUR OWN INTERESTS *FIRST*

Before you ever consider a serious relationship, develop your own interests *first*, then you can seek women in those interests. Surprise! When you both have something in common besides lust, the relationship might last longer than a fever. It might even develop into a friendship, which lasts longer than a wilted corsage from the homecoming dance or the senior prom. Tiger Woods may have been better served seeking out a fellow golfer or a professional athlete who understood his fast-lane lifestyle and pressures instead of a Swedish au pair.

RULE NO. 3:
DANCE BEFORE YOU DATE

Take social dance, Argentine tango, East Coast swing, country western swing, or cotillion—preferably before you've had a single date. First, you will learn that holding a woman close doesn't mean it is true love. You have to hold her close if you are going to lead her in couples' dancing. But more important, you will learn to treat a woman with respect and courtesy. It's much easier to learn the right way to do things when you start than to unlearn bad habits later.

RULE NO. 4:
UNDERSTAND THE LAW OF SINE CURVES

This is the dating behavior of the average woman, as explained by the mathematical concept known as the sine curve (see the diagrams that follow).

The Sine Curve

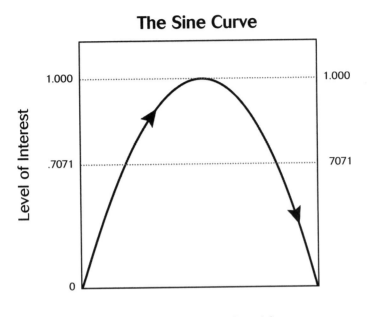

Time in the Relationship

When the sine curve begins at zero, the average woman becomes interested in a guy. Her increased interest is depicted on the y-axis, the time in the relationship by the x-axis.

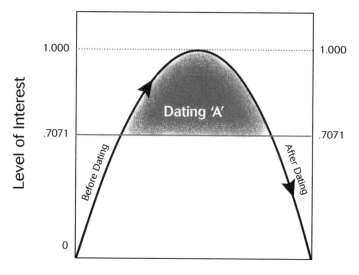

Time in the Relationship

Over time, her interest in a guy will increase to the threshold of dating him. At this point, interest is measured as 0.7071 on the sine curve. From this point on, the woman and the guy are a couple.

The slope of the sine curve is positive until it peaks at 1.0000, reflecting the upside of any dating relationship. When the sine curve reaches 1.0000, there is both good news and bad news for the happy couple. The measurement of 1.0000 represents the apex of the relationship. Both partners are satisfied with the relationship at this point in time. But sadly, after this, the relationship loses momentum. At 1.0000 things will never be so good again.

The Sine Curve

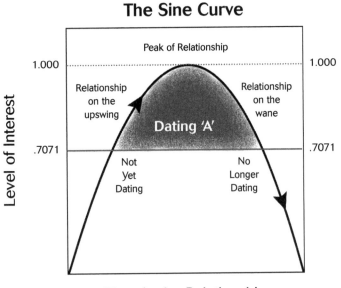

Many a romantic looks back at his or her broken relationship and yearns for the 1.000 moment, which can be approximated at a homecoming or prom dance, a special time together, or a romantic weekend. Although the couple is still together, one or both know something isn't right. At this moment many guys don't see what is coming next. But there is no malice involved in the unfortunate downside of the sine curve. It is a phenomenon of dating.

For men to grasp the Law of the Sine Curve, they must understand one important concept: *most women do not like to be alone.* There are formal dances, holiday and family get-togethers, club or sorority functions, and Friday and Saturday nights that demand a male escort. They simply need somebody to be that guy, the dutiful boyfriend, and if they have decided you don't make the cut for the part-time or permanent position, they'll begin to look elsewhere for suitable candidates. They may still be dating you, but that loving feeling is slipping away. At this point the average girl will begin to look for other potential partners to replace the current number one, whose slope is now becoming increasingly negative. As the sine curve again reaches 0.7071, the relationship is again at the threshold of dating/not dating, otherwise known as "breaking up." You may not know it at the time, but when the relationship has long since peaked, then she will break up with you. Unfortunately, many men in mirage relationships don't see 0.7071 coming. They aren't able to feel the obvious negative feelings the woman has been experiencing for a while.

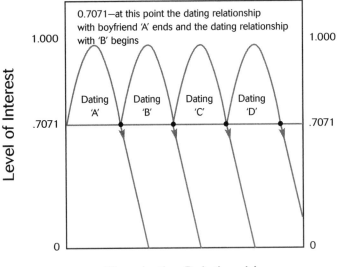

Level of Interest

1.000

.7071

0.7071—at this point the dating relationship with boyfriend 'A' ends and the dating relationship with 'B' begins

Dating 'A' Dating 'B' Dating 'C' Dating 'D'

1.000

.7071

0

Time in the Relationship

Popular and skillful women will have several future sine curves to cultivate, even as they date another guy. As they end one relationship at the negative end of 0.7071, they will have another guy at the threshold of dating on the positive side of 0.7071 on another sine curve. Thus, the woman can theoretically never be without an escort if she carefully ends one sine curve and begins another.

This woman will never miss a homecoming dance or prom. Why should she? Dating should be kept as a tool to determine compatibility, not to pretend you've found your soul mate for life. Rushing into a serious physical relationship with someone you barely know (becoming "joined at the hip") leads to possessive relationships with guys who don't know how to bow out gracefully. Women *should* date with the sine curve, and guys *should* expect it and not resent it. If both partners are not satisfied with a dating relationship, they should be free to leave it at any time without guilt. But artificial intimacy is often used by men in mirage relationships to make women feel too guilty to leave floundering relationships.

RULE NO. 5: NO KISSING OR HUGGING ON THE FIRST DATE

It sounds puritanical and oppressive, but this rule is keeping in line with the theme of this book—getting to know someone before becoming physically involved with them. Dating should be used to help determine compatibility, not for the cheap thrill of artificial intimacy. Can a heterosexual male make a clear intellectual determination of the suitability of temperaments after a tender good-night kiss? Don't delude yourselves—it's impossible! Many are the men who have rationalized a relationship based on physical attraction, only to wind up committed to someone who makes them feel completely miserable. So give yourself the opportunity to soberly judge a first date and the potential for a mutually satisfying relationship. One simply cannot weigh the pros and cons when one is punch-drunk on physical intimacy.

Men are drawn to the physical anyway. Rob, a twenty-five-year-old grad student, was dating a beautiful blond beyond his wildest dreams. But her personality was definitely a "plain Jane." Rob finally was able to step back and analyze that they had one thing in common, and it wasn't a mutual love of University of Alabama football. To marry her would be to commit himself to a life of Chinese water torture. There would be no compatibility and, at best, a messy, expensive divorce. Like Rob, one should save oneself the grief of diving headfirst into relationships that are only centimeters deep. Use first dates to explore the potential for a relationship. If things are right for both of you, there will be plenty of time for sweet affection later.

RULE NO. 6:
AVOID THE PROM SYNDROME

Spend money on your dates in proportion to the number of months you have seen each other. There is a senseless trend going on in the dating world. Men lavishly entertain on the first few dates and formal dances like the prom, at a truly unsustainable level to bedazzle their women. Since they aren't going to use a limousine as the family car once they marry and have children, why do men spend hundreds of dollars renting one for a formal dance? Limos are more than a mobile party that allows one to drink and ride legally—plenty of sober Mormon kids are renting them along with the party-hearty kids. It's all about excess and performing to expectations.

Society approves of such ostentatious displays in the romantic world. It is a bold economic display of class with a hidden catch. By lavishly spending on the date or dance, there is incredible pressure for the date to culminate in the ultimate romantic fantasy. Throw compatibility out the window—all that matters is a "happy" ending for this five-hour drama. If either partner has legitimate reservations about the relationship, they are pressured to deny them for the evening lest they be the party pooper. This phenomenon has grown worse and worse over the last twenty years, where the current high school boy faces a price tag of up to $1,000 for his prom (limo, tuxedo, corsage, pictures, expensive candlelight dinner, dance tickets, hotel room, etc.). This lavish prom display is merely artificial intimacy at record levels of practice in our society.

A remedy for this insanity is simple. If you meet someone at school, spend time talking to her as you walk to class. Invite her to a group activity where you can interact freely with no pressure. See how she gets along with your friends. If a real friendship develops, go together to public activities like the football game, the beach, or the park as you would with your male friends. Real relationships grow without someone forcing them to accelerate through artificial intimacy. Only go to inexpensive restaurants or coffeehouses to meet, so the emphasis is on the conversation. Date sensibly and inexpensively.

RULE NO. 7: GIVE THE RELATIONSHIP TIME TO DEVELOP

Men feel pressure to "close the deal" before another guy comes along to sweep their intended love away. That is based on ignorance. If a woman likes you, she will not be swept away by another unless she thinks you aren't interested. So much goes into the decision a woman makes about who she is attracted to and who isn't her type. If you are the right one for her, there isn't much you have to do. Just be yourself and give her the opportunity to get to know you and decide if she accepts the real you. That is the ultimate goal of healthy dating: to find someone who accepts your naked self.

We have known people who dated in a healthy manner and met their future mate early in life. But for most of us, the average dating relationship will end far short of marriage, so expect it. Don't be shocked when every overture isn't reciprocated. Remember the Law of the Sine Curve: if she sours on you, then it was never meant to be anyway. You just hit the down slope of 0.7071, as we all have. Let the disappointment, shame, and control go. Do not believe the Hollywood myth that "no means yes" and that persistence will wear down a woman's resistance, like *Seinfeld's* persistent mirage man George Costanza. Respect a woman's right to not choose you. Don't blame yourself if you don't connect with a woman to whom you are strongly attracted. Accept the disconnect as a natural part of the dating process and move on! There are millions of women in this world to meet.

RULE NO. 8: FOUR-HOUR PHONE CALLS DO NOT MEAN A THING

Quality matters over the length of your talks both on the phone and in person. Men can be fooled into thinking that they are connecting, when in truth, it may be that the woman is polite and skillful. When you date a woman, check her reactions. Are you carrying the conversation, or is she? Discounting for nervousness, the healthy man must determine if the woman has potential for a friendship.

If the woman is doing all the talking about herself, it can be a sign of self-centeredness, which will wear thin for most men over the long haul. Marty, a thirty-one-year-old fireman, could literally walk away from the phone while his girlfriend was talking and she wouldn't notice for several minutes. To her, a relationship was someone to dump on. We would ask Marty how his latest conversation with Chatty Cathy went: "Was her percentage of talking to you 99 percent to 1 percent, 95 percent to 5 percent, 90 percent to 10 percent, or 80 percent to 20 percent?" Any of the four answers is a loser relationship. But many desperate men like Marty settle for this type of woman who couldn't care less how they are doing as long as they have a pulse and can nod at the appropriate moment to convey rapt attention.

If a first date starts out with either you or her doing most of the talking, that isn't necessarily bad. Someone has to talk and leave the nervousness behind. Use her talkativeness to find out about her background, including her family, to see if you share similar experiences and outlooks on the world. Likewise, if you are doing most of the talking, try to use your experiences as springboard topics to get her to talk about herself. The idea is to move beyond the superficial to gain some real insight into her personality and character.

Eventually, a good conversation resembles a tennis match, where both partners serve and volley. But some conversations may appear to be going well but lack a vital ingredient essential to a healthy relationship: interest. If her curiosity is not piqued about your background, family, interests, and goals, you aren't connecting, even if you talk on the phone for four hours. She may merely be an excellent conversationalist who can talk to anybody. If she is truly interested in you as a friend, she should want to know more about you besides your favorite foods. It should be gradual, but each time you talk for an extended period, there should be a growing knowledge and interest shared between each of you. There is no future in someone who doesn't genuinely care about the real you behind the sunglasses.

RULE NO. 9: THERE IS NO HONEYMOON

Remember, the fourth step is that the honeymoon is a myth. If you think things will get better in the future with your woman, you are wrong. Relationships are hard to find, hard to maintain, and are vulnerable to many internal and external pressures. If you do not feel comfortable dating a particular woman, please articulate it to her and seek counseling if you both wish to save the relationship. Otherwise you should consider ending the relationship. Never "do someone a favor" by staying in a dating liaison that is on the down slope of 0.7071. Please don't be passive and let it degenerate slowly. That is to live in the realm of the unfeeling mirage man.

Barnes & Noble is full of books on relationships, but most men erroneously think a relationship comes naturally, like a baseball swing. Furthermore, the universe is against a relationship maintaining a healthy, steady state indefinitely. Relationships are likewise easier to dismantle than maintain. Expect relationships to seize like a car engine if neglected. As a feeling, healthy man, you must risk the end of the relationship by confronting the truth if things have changed between you.

RULE NO. 10: WRITE A LETTER TO END A CASUAL DATING RELATIONSHIP

Write a letter? "Why don't you tell me to my face you're leaving now?" you scream. Well, the point is to have some type of closure besides not calling anymore. If you prefer a face-to-face confrontation where physical attraction can sway noble intentions—then go, brave and strong soldier! If you prefer the telephone call as an indirect-direct confrontation where physical contact is limited but emotional contact is unrestricted, go to it. We urge some kind of ending as a token of respect for the person you have gotten to know.

If you have dated as a means of determining compatibility and have found this dating partner wanting, there should be some difficulty ending the liaison. The physical presence of a woman is intoxicating. Her perfume, her sparkling eyes, her naughty smile, the curve in her calf . . . well, we could go on and on, but the point is, women have a powerful pull on men. Presidents Kennedy and Clinton risked their political careers for their desire for women. Great men throughout history have met their demise over a Delilah, Bathsheba, or Monica. So never discount the fact that the healthy man can be overcome by the sweet cologne of femininity. Take it into account as a factor if you are unsure of ending a relationship. It is often the only thing that keeps you dating her. That is why the healthy man never cuts himself off from his friends and family (see Stage 3 in Chapter 7). Use your trusted friends as devil's advocates to see if your judgment is swayed by sexual attraction. If you can determine that the liaison does not have a future that includes compatibility, you must end the relationship. Please do it with the respect all women deserve. Let her know in person, by phone, or written word that things did not work out. We've provided a sample letter that follows as a guide, if you need it.

Sample Letter Ending a Casual Dating Relationship

Date: _____

Dear _____,

I wanted to write to thank you for the nice time together. I really enjoyed getting to know you. I think you are a beautiful woman with tremendous talents that will take you far in life. However, I feel that we do not share enough in common to be anything more than just friends. If you would like to continue as friends, I would enjoy that. But if you would prefer to see other people given your busy schedule, I will understand.

Again, it has been great getting to know you. Take care.

Your friend,

The most effective means of ending a relationship is the written word rather than doing so in person or on the phone. First, it saves the other person, as well as you, the embarrassment of an awkward scene. Some people do not take bad news as well as others. Even though the healthy man may date in an emotionally open and honest way, his dating partner may misinterpret things or get her hopes up for something that is not going to come to pass. He cannot be responsible for her reaction, only his. The letter gives the woman some time to digest the news before a phone call or personal visit occurs, so things will be less emotional.

The written word is a good tool for the mirage man in recovery. Despite his best motives, the newly emerging healthy man is human and may have behaved poorly or mis-led his dating partner inadvertently. He may be learning new, healthy ways of relating to women but still stumbles into deception. The written word gives a recovering man a tool to confront the truth and return to health. For many mirage men in recovery, confrontation is the hardest thing after a life of deception. Through a letter one can calmly and clearly state the reason for ending the dating relationship with honesty and respect. Knowing this tool is available, healthy men can date with honesty and not go through the fear and mind games of "letting someone down easy" or avoiding her.

Whatever method of communication, please avoid using voice mail or an answering machine to end a relationship. It is the worst of all ways; you hear their voice yet are denied any response, and the messages are improvised and rushed. If you end a relationship, do it as you would have them do it to you: gently, well thought out and expressed, and done with class.

12

HEALING
THE MIRAGE MAN

"Honestly, I think I can do better.
My marriage is only going to help me.
I found a person I can talk to and a person
who is going to be by my side through
thick and thin. Elin has instilled a
lot of confidence in me in
all aspects of my life."[1]

—*Tiger Woods, April 19, 2005*

*T**his book has good news for* the mirage couple. Even though your marriage may be based on deceit, it can be healed. Even Tiger Woods's marriage can be healed. The solution is based on a search for the true man behind the mask and a new relationship based on honesty. Let's look at each aspect of healing the mirage relationship in detail.

IN SEARCH OF THE TRUE MAN

We can find mirage men searching for solutions to their miserable marriages all over America. Tired of the effects of the deceptive life they have created for themselves, they seek help in therapy, 12-step support groups, Promise Keepers rallies, and men's movement retreats. Few of these same men arrive at these venues of help purely of their own volition. They are sent by their fed-up wives, who no longer respect their mirage men and find their characteristic spewing resentment and addictive behavior tearing their marriages apart.

You might observe one of these men standing up at a support group meeting, sheepishly explaining that he doesn't know why his wife sent him. In the next breath he'll tell you that he has to keep another set of clothes in his SUV in case the wife throws him out of the house for the weekend (as usual). You wince as he tells his story of how he was so in love once, but now his marriage hangs by a thread. Again and again he complains that his wife doesn't want to hear the truth about her dishonest husband, that she just wants his addictive behavior to stop. But there is no quick fix. His resentment and compulsive behaviors are symptomatic of deep-seated hurt and anger that are not amenable to the Band-Aid healing approach so common in these times.

Healing for the mirage man takes more than a couple of Promise Keepers retreats, emergency meetings with former President Clinton's three spiritual advisors, or court-ordered therapy over the telephone (à la O. J. Simpson). The key to any real healing for the mirage man is in his rediscovery of the true self, thought for so long to not be presentable to anyone, especially his wife. This process must include a return to the painful days of childhood that most men spend a lifetime avoiding and overcoming through achievement. Yet it was these early traumas that convinced him he was not "good enough" by himself and not worthy of love.

As we learned in the earlier chapter on approval seeking, boys learn to disconnect from their feelings early in life. In their elementary school years, they learn to deny their feelings in the name of manhood. By adolescence, a boy has been conditioned to put up with anything to achieve his goals. With this deadening of emotions nearly complete, the boy faces the special challenge of approaching adolescence: attempting to find a safe haven in a social clique.

Adolescence for the American male is one continuous attempt at protection by losing the true self in other roles. These roles have a permanent disfiguring effect. Young men lose touch with their true tastes after years of adapting to the prescribed tastes of the clique. The phony roles of adolescence are often so effective in protecting one from harm that they become as familiar to the young man as his clothes. Why leave something that served him so well for so long in those painful and dangerous "Wonder Years"?

If the deception did not sabotage interpersonal relationships in adulthood, there would be few indeed that would ever shed this useful macho armor of childhood. But successful heterosexual relations for the mirage man are impossible without this difficult transition back to the true self.

By returning to the painful early years, the mirage man will be able to see that he is not alone in his behavior. Many males never let go of the defense mechanism of deception that helped them survive the anything goes world of male childhood and adolescence. By an honest appraisal of his early life, the mirage man can slowly work toward the present. By discovering the root causes of his present resentment and addictive behavior, the recovering mirage man can seek specific professional help for his individual character defects. All through this long-term process, the mirage man must fight the natural urge to avoid the painful self-revelations and retreat back into his chronic, sick condition. Given the amount of time spent in the deceptive lifestyle, it is easy to see why many men give up the journey toward wholeness.

Once the mirage man's character defects and compulsive behavior are brought to the light, he must decide whether he wants to continue with them or seek healing for each ingrained aspect of his chronic condition. It may seem obvious that once the mirage man becomes aware of his sick behavior he would want to cease it, but many people find their medicating behaviors to be as familiar and comforting

as an old friend. Professional help should be sought in dealing with these huge obstacles to healing, including intensive
clinical treatment of specific compulsive behaviors like sex
addiction. Trained mental health care specialists should be
consulted to diagnose the extent of the mirage man's psychological problems and any physical contribution to them like
depression, hypoglycemia, and so on. Then support groups in
the 12-step tradition can aid in the long-term healing of
codependency and other specific addictions. For instance, the
12-Step support group Sexaholics Anonymous (SA) would
provide daily support for the recovering addict. In addition to
daily and weekly meetings that stress anonymity, SA pro-
vides a "sponsor" or a personal contact for those willing to
take the baby steps necessary to restore a healthy sexuality.[2]

Needless to say, the mirage man can spend years working
his way through the recovery process to find his true self.
There are courageous women who will wait patiently for the
worm of a mirage man to morph into an honest butterfly.
However, there is a great challenge to both partners once the
mirage man has sought and received healing.

A NEW RELATIONSHIP BASED ON HONESTY

The mirage man must risk the loss of his unhealthy relationships as he begins a radically new lifestyle of sharing his true feelings, needs, and goals with his mate and friends. Switching from a life of deception to rigorous honesty is the only way to avoid a relapse into the comfortable sickness of the old ways of dealing with people.

Support groups are a safe place for the recovering mirage man to try brand-new, healthy ways of relating to others. The strict rules and healthy boundaries practiced in the support group allow the man to risk honesty without being slammed. Then he can slowly try to incorporate the new honesty in his marriage and friendships in the harsh real world. But be warned—learning to take the risk of being honest takes a long time to master for those whose dishonest manner is a natural reflex from childhood. Furthermore, honesty is rarely warmly received by a spouse who has grown accustomed to the mirage man's approval-seeking ways. Many mirage men are genuinely shocked when their wife rejects the unveiling of their true self. The desire to avoid confrontations with the wife through continued deception will be powerful. Mistakes will be made, but encouragement from male support groups will help the sincerely contrite man on his way to a new honesty in his relationships.

Please understand how threatening change can be to the mirage man's wife. The prospect of having one's predictable (if miserable) life thrown into chaos and an uncertain future often results in a strong backlash by a spouse who only wanted incremental change in a few areas. Often the wife only wanted the deceptive man to cease his serial adultery or out-of-control alcoholism and return to that pliable approval seeker of courtship.

Some don't ever want to acknowledge the truth that their marriage was a sham of deception from the start. Consider the letter to Ann Landers from "Silently Weeping in Kansas," who was shocked to find out upon her husband's sudden death that he was a prolific sex addict. Her advice to married men was not to deal with their deceptive behavior, *but to get rid of the evidence so your grieving wives won't have to deal with it after you are gone!*[3]

However much they may insist to the contrary on daytime talk shows, many wives of mirage men would rather continue in fantasyland than meet their husband's true self face-to-face. Not knowing what their husband is truly like and how he really feels moment to moment is preferable to many women unprepared for the truth lurking behind their husband's baby blue eyes.[4]

Some women *are* threatened by the loss of the mirage relationship. They are suddenly challenged to a new level of honesty in their marriage. Many of the women's character defects and addictive behavior may begin to become noticeable after years of submersion to the more glaring inadequacies of the deceptive husband. A comfortable enabling by the wife will suddenly be exposed as the sick contribution to the mirage man's pathological behavior. No one likes to think of themselves as practicing bad behavior, so some wives will refuse to look at their responsibility in perpetuating the Tiger Woods Syndrome and the need for their own resentments and addictions to be dealt with. If women's magazines are any indication, there are a significant number of women who would rather focus on what type of affair their husband is having (Dr. Bonnie Eaker Weil lists five different types in her book!) than accept the fact that their relationship has been unhealthy from day one. That involves an acceptance of some responsibility.

To truly change a relationship from deceptive to healthy, the mirage man must be willing to risk the end of the marriage or cohabitation by practicing honesty and candor. He can no longer redefine the meaning of the word *is*, wait until he is forced to admit his behavior, or omit what he knows is the truth. The mirage man must "hit bottom" in terms of continuing the deceptive life. Unless he truly believes he has nowhere to go but to health, he will slide back to his old, familiar, political ways exhibited by Bill Clinton, Eliot Spitzer, Mark Sanford, John Edwards, Newt Gingrich, and Gary Condit. If he still believes he has the option of practicing "a kinder, gentler" version of deceit, he will mend it instead of ending it. But a "mended" mirage relationship only buys time. The core issues of two incompatible lovers cannot be smoothed over with sweet talk, promises, and second honeymoons. Unless the mirage man ends his deceptive behavior, he will remain in a terminal relationship of resigned compliance, reaping brokenness and destruction.

This book has been written to heal existing marriages, not to give license to men to junk their wives and lovers for new "healthy" partners. The hope is that once a wife knows her husband is cognizant of his deception and wishes to change, she will embrace her husband's recovery and support his growth. The immediate reality is that the recovering mirage man should not expect gratitude but instead anger, tears, alienation, and opposition from his wife.

The contrite mirage man needs to continually reassure her that he is changing his life out of love and concern for her. He needs to also keep in mind that his wife may feel cheated out of an emotionally satisfying relationship by her thief of hearts. She should be resentful and distrusting! She must deal with the truth that she has been deceived, wasting years of her life on a mirage. She needs constant comforting that this isn't just another scam by a proven con artist.

The mirage man needs to share his true self, even if his wife is initially unreceptive. She must be given plenty of time and space to deal with the fact that she was deceived and now must start a new relationship from scratch. This may be too much for her to deal with, and she may wish to end the marriage. The mirage man must understand the real possibility that his wife may reject his true self and file for divorce. That is her choice, and the healthy man will let her finally choose her mate with no subterfuge.

This is the crisis that couples like Tiger Woods and Elin Nordegren faced. If the wife chooses to stay in the marriage, she must be informed that every assumption about the old unhealthy relationship must be challenged.

This remodeling process can be an exciting opportunity for the couple if they have the love and courage to start from scratch. Too many people prefer to build a house of love on a cracked slab rather than excavate the ruined stone and lay down new concrete. One must establish a new foundation consisting of honesty to build a healthy relationship between a man and a woman. Enlist the help of a proven marital therapist as you begin the rebuilding effort. Intensive marital counseling is recommended as the man seeks healing from the Tiger Woods Syndrome, because his changes affect his wife so profoundly. The true man will emerge from a healing process that will be long and arduous. The couple must keep the faith that the reward of an emotionally satisfying romance for both partners is worth the painful price of acknowledgment and rebuilding.

13

SLIP SLIDING AWAY AND THE SERIAL CHEATER

"To go against the dominant
thinking of your friends, of most of
the people you see everyday, is
perhaps the most difficult act
of heroism you can have."

—Theodore H. White
American political writer (1915–1986)

*M*en suffering from the Tiger Woods Syndrome attend therapy and support groups meetings to deal with the inevitable side effects of their lifestyle. The wash-out rate, unfortunately, is quite high. Many men eventually tire of the challenge to become healthy and retreat to the comfortable mire of deception.

The reasons for relapsing are varied. For some, the fear of abandonment erodes their will to change no matter how sick and degrading the deceptive relationship has become. They would rather not risk the loss of a flawed but known relationship and end up alone.

Other men abandon recovery because they fear they might provoke their wife to legal action and their subsequent financial ruin. For Craig, a forty-five-year-old businessman, the choice is a monetary one: better to stay sick and flush than healthy and fleeced by divorce lawyers, alimony, and child support payments. He will spend the rest of his life seeing how much of his resentment and addictions he can safely express before his wife reaches the crisis point again. Men like this live life on the edge of divorce cliff.

Some men, like Tom, a twenty-eight-year-old teacher, dabble in the knowledge of recovery and attempt to learn a boundary skill here or a communication tip there without ever renouncing their destructive lifestyle. They may add the role of "healthy hubby" to their repertoire of deceptive roles.

Tragically, some men who initially seek healing after the end of one mirage relationship will insanely begin another with someone they meet in their therapy group, thinking that somehow things will be different this time with a new partner. In 12-Step lore, this is known as "13th Stepping." Armed with a little knowledge of boundaries and codependency, they plunge into a new romance just as structurally sick as the last one. They never accept the hard truth that one of the chief causes of all their poor relationships with women has been their deceptive ways. These men demonize their old lovers and wives and delude themselves with the notion that it is always the woman's fault when their relationships end. They like to tell people they are "unlucky at love" and absolve themselves of all responsibility for the trail of tears they leave behind.

Is it any wonder *Time* magazine runs a cover photo of a pig with the caption "Are Men Really That Bad?"[1] These various "villains" just listed in the preceding paragraphs are culled from our experiences with men seeking help! These are men who at least sensed something was wrong and tried to do the right thing for themselves and their partners. Imagine the quality of men who stay submerged in the sickness of the syndrome their whole lives. But what of the married man who honors his commitment to his wife and children? Here is a guy who is doing the right thing. Shouldn't the outcome be better for the man who tries to preserve the building block of America, the family unit?

Unfortunately, the long-term prognosis for the married mirage man is poor. As the man lives out his life based on deception, he grows bitter toward his wife and family. He realizes he is doomed to spend his life with a woman he doesn't really like. He knows he must spend countless hours doing things he doesn't like to do to continue his phony role or else risk the end of the relationship. He knows she will be disillusioned with him when she finally realizes he isn't Mr. Sensitive. Physical affection as harmless as hand-holding or a hug will become rare. The mirage man will seek to medicate his accumulating resentment and pain he feels through addictive behavior. Workaholism, religion, serial adultery, gossip, food, sports, television, power, alcohol and drugs are just a few of the ways the mirage man will compulsively anesthetize his feelings.

In the resigned compliance stage, the man will become more and more emotionally unavailable to his wife and family as his addictions take their long term toll on him. At this point many men feel trapped in the relationship due to the commitments yet fear leaving because of the monetary and emotional cost of divorce. They will live a dual life as serial cheaters.

SERIAL ADULTERERS

What do many men who practice serial adultery want? Therapist and author Marvin Allen gives us insight:

❖

Many men tell me that they feel a deep sense of connection with their sexual partners. Most of the time they must feel cut off from people. Sex can create an instant connection. For a few passionate moments they feel united with another person body and soul. For many of the thousands of men I have talked to, sex can be a spiritual, almost religious experience. It's one of the rare opportunities they have to feel truly alive.[2]

The problem with the unfaithful mirage man using sex as a means of connecting with another human being is that it lasts for only a few fleeting hours before the serial cheater must flee back to his alternate universe where he lives the life as husband, provider, and father. The next day the mirage man will find himself just as alone and disconnected to his unsuspecting spouse and children as before. This can feed the need to keep seeing the person who gives him the temporary high, connection, and escape from reality.

What serial adulterers are seeking is the unconditional acceptance of the naked self. It is certainly satisfying at one level to connect with another human being but there is an empty feeling after the passionate interlude when the mirage man realizes his wife doesn't even know him. The mirage man can pretend the women he picks up in bars accept him unconditionally even though the relationships are purely based on physical attraction and charm.

Simon, a thirty-three-year-old hotel chain executive,

spoke of how he felt such condemnation from his wife whenever he tried to express any of his true self. He had deceived her during their initial courtship into believing he was her Prince Charming, so she logically bristled whenever he deviated from the script. Simon felt less and less satisfaction in his marriage and sought acceptance in the arms of virtual strangers. He said that at least with the women he picked up in bars and restaurants while on the road, he could pretend that they accepted him unconditionally during the lovemaking. He had ceased to feel any acceptance from his disillusioned wife.

Mirage men crave acceptance, even if it just for one night. There is symbolic physical nakedness in a sexual encounter, even though it is but a diversion from the terrible reality that no one in the world truly knows and accepts them. That is why so many "happily married" men seek one-night stands at hotel bars and enjoy lap dances at sleazy strip joints. They have become so desperate they are willing to pretend with women they would have been ashamed to be seen with during high school.

Mirage men are not finding acceptance in their conventional monogamous relationships. They practice denial in the early stages of a mirage relationship by pretending that their partner is accepting their naked self. The reality is that their relationship is based on inappropriate emotional and physical intimacy and the deception of approval seeking. There is symbolic physical nakedness in each sexual encounter, but for a mirage man, there is no acceptance of the naked self because the rejection-fearing mirage man never gives his partner the chance to really know and accept him.

Mirage men usually won't admit there is a serious problem in their marriage until they reach a crisis point. Many will cope by practicing serial cheating in their marriage and others will employ women to provide them with the temporary acceptance they find lacking in their steady relationships. It's an ugly picture indeed and it won't change until these men begin to recognize their complicity in creating unsatisfying relationships with women that leave them aching for more.

Needless to say, the future for the mirage man is grim. He will experience little joy in his conventional life and his children will learn to stay clear of him when he is emotionally hung-over. He may try to remain superficially cheerful (especially at work) but his smile is a mask used to keep his family at arm's length so his seething true self doesn't make an unexpected appearance. He may try to be technically perfect in his role of husband-provider so that he will be spared criticism, much like a child excels in sports or studies just to avoid the parent's critical eye. He will tend to avoid wife-instigated discussions about current problems in the marriage and family to keep the light of introspection from revealing his complicity in the mirage relationship.

The mirage man's addictions will lead to an exaggeration of his character defects. He will become a caricature of his early Mr. Sensitive character. His family will learn to adjust as he becomes more and more eccentric, after years of living with no moorings to his true self. Resentment may inspire him to occasional out-of-character blow ups that will shock and amaze those who thought they knew him. This will spawn dysfunctional behavior in his children who look up to him as a prototypical male. His daughters will tend to seek emotionally unavailable mates like him and his sons will model his deceptive behavior in relating to girls. His family will perpetuate his sickness to new generations.

The mirage man's marriage will continue its gradual downward spiral as the years pass. His wife will tire of a man she can dominate but not respect. She may numb herself with addictions so she can tolerate existence with her resentful, emotionally numb partner. Over time, these addictions may not provide enough anesthetic to put up with her husband's antics. She may forsake creature comforts for the chance at romance with someone who appears from a distance to be superior to her uncommunicative slug of a husband. Thirty or forty years into her marriage she may sue for divorce and take a chance on love again.

LEAVING THE MIRAGE MAN

Some women leave their mirage men in the latter days of marriage. That is for the adventurous woman willing to risk her children's wrath, her sure retirement and her social standing for a chance at happiness. Others awaken to the sad state of affairs and demand radical changes within the structure of the marriage.

Why do middle-aged women wait so long? The poor quality of the mirage marriage may be hidden from view for years as the couple distracts themselves with the hustle and bustle of raising a family on double incomes. When the kids leave home and retirement nears, the long-standing problems of the couple become too much to ignore. Wendy Crisp, spokeswoman for the National Association of Female Executives, describes this day of reckoning:

❖

"If you never really liked each other or have nothing to share, you have to basically reach agreements that a significant portion of your time will be spent doing separate things . . . Separate things could mean separate bedrooms.[3]

When the mirage man reaches the crisis phase of the resigned compliance state, this is often the ironic scenario. The mirage man originally deceived the woman into a relationship to get sex and companionship. Over the years, the couple discovers they don't like each other and have nothing to share. The final act of the deceptive man's life may feature him living in a romantic Siberia, whiling away his Golden Years exiled from the marriage bed. He and his wife live together with nothing in common except children, grandchildren, and a long-simmering mutual resentment of one another.

The thought of wasting one's life in such a relational hell should encourage us all to think twice before submitting to our society's mutated method of modern love. The good news is we have a choice: do we perpetuate this romantic cancer on our partner and children, or do we become part of the cure? We believe that the life-affirming wisdom of this book will lead thoughtful men and women back into relationships of true intimacy.

14

HOW COMPATIBLE WILL WE BE?

"The art of life is to show your hand.
There is no diplomacy like candor.
You may lose by it now and then,
but it will be a loss well gained if you do.
Nothing is so boring as having to
keep up a deception."

—E. V. Lucas, English author and critic (1868–1938)

We have explored the destructive nature of the Tiger Woods Syndrome in detail. The union of a man and a woman based on deception leads to loneliness and heartbreak. We have pointed the way to recognizing the deceptive relationship and the way toward healing for the mirage man and his wife. Now we are ready to propose an alternative, healthy relationship. This healthy relationship model can be used by young men who wish to begin dating as well as older men who have turned their backs on the deceptive methods of this age. This model should also be studied by women so that they will demand better from their men.

The beginning of health in romance must be based on a revolutionary form of dating. By that we mean a form of courtship dating back to the days after the Revolutionary War. According to historian Ellen Rothman, "For both men and women, the best defense against deception was openness. After the turn of the [nineteenth] century, openness became almost an obsession for courting couples. In the nineteenth century, it was no longer enough to be sincere in one's affections; lovers were urged to be frank and open about everything."[1]

Imagine if today's men used this revolutionary concept of candor. Our society would be strengthened with healthy relationships. Instead of desperately searching for somebody to accept his romantic overtures, the healthy man would defer his need for instant gratification and use the dating process to select likely partners among those women of compatible temperament and like interests.

As one can tell from a quick glance at the television, this is in direct opposition to the current trend in American society. American men have been encouraged to look to any woman above their minimum standard of beauty who will accept them as a potential mate. To practice healthy dating, men must resist this siren song of sensuality that "all that matters is getting it on." Dating should be used like a scalpel, to slice through the extraneous and superficial to reach the significant other.

To be able to date in a healthy, revolutionary manner, a twenty-first-century man must first establish his own identity apart from any other person. Until he understands his own feelings, needs, and goals, he will be incapable of establishing a healthy relationship with a woman. The natural desire to seek approval from another human being to gain acceptance, coupled with the potent nectar of sexual attraction, will lead even men seeking recovery back into their toxic habits. One must enter the dating game with a definite goal in mind: to opt for a relationship with compatible temperaments and significant common interests. To settle for anything less is to sell out.

FINDING COMPATIBILITY

Compatibility is a very elusive goal for the man who chooses to date in a healthy manner. He must take into account that many physically desirable women are extremely difficult to get along with once the thrill of artificial intimacy dissipates. To date in a healthy manner, the man must assume that his own compatibility problems will inevitably surface once the newness of the relationship fades into the harsh reality of day-to-day existence. Consider the sad testimony of Academy Award–winning actress Halle Berry, fresh from a messy divorce from Atlanta Braves and New York Yankees outfielder David Justice: "I've learned so much through marriage—and I've learned that, the next time around, I'm going to take the time to find out, 'Do I really like you?' Not 'Do I love you and am in love and do I lust after you,' but 'Do I like who you are, and can I laugh with you and play with you?' I think I might take the time to figure that out."[2]

To avoid romantic involvement with someone of clashing temperaments, like Berry endured with Justice, one needs to see past the physical attraction and charm. Think of the work or school acquaintances that you initially liked but proved to be incompatible with as time wore on. Likewise, in romance one must exert the discipline to see beyond attractive features to the potential partner's compatibility with your personality style.

How does one objectively evaluate a potential partner's personality to see if there is hope for long-term compatibility? Psychological experts have compiled indexes of personality style. We suggest using one that denotes four general personality types: analytical, driven, expressive, and amiable:

1. **Analytical:** thoughtful, organized, quiet, and high-achieving, but also overly critical, humorless, and boring at times.

2. **Driven:** self-assured, innovative, self-motivated,

stimulating, and good leaders, but also manipulative, unsympathetic, impatient, and domineering.

3. **Expressive:** exciting, funny, and charming people who are also talkative, low-achieving, needy, and sometimes flaky.

4. **Amiable:** even-tempered, friendly, moderately organized, and agreeable, but also indecisive, resistant to change, and uncommunicative when troubled.

Each personality type has its positive aspects and its negative aspects. For example, the analytical and the amiable are less assertive, while the driven and the expressive are more assertive. Do you like someone who stands up for his rights, or are you embarrassed when he causes a scene when his steak is undercooked or the airline lost his reservation?

The analytical and driven are less emotional, while the amiable and expressive are more emotional. Would you rather hang out with someone who lets you know how he is really feeling, or are you repelled by someone who wears his emotions on his sleeve? These are important factors in deciding who you would wish to date, much less spend the rest of your life with. Given your own range of emotion and assertiveness in your personality, you will connect with certain personality types and clash with others. Let's take a closer look at each personality type.

You may be attracted to the expressive personality type, because they are exciting, funny, and charming people. However, expressives tend to be talkative, low-achieving, needy, and—worst of all—flaky. If needing someone you can depend on overshadows the fun qualities of the expressive personality, you may react by choosing to date the reliable but introverted analytical personality.

The analytical personality type tends to be thoughtful, organized, quiet, and high-achieving. That can be a good antidote to a bad experience with a flaky, expressive personality type. However, the analytical personality also has the negative tendencies of being overly critical, skeptical, humorless, and boring. You may react to the critical nature of the analytical person by dating a person who is amiable.

The amiable personality type is even-tempered, friendly, moderately organized, and agreeable. What a relief after the last analytical person, right? Unfortunately, the amiable also tend to be indecisive, resent change, and will not tell you when they are troubled. The amiable person's poor communication skills and lack of goals may then send you for relief to a driven person.

The driven personality type is self-assured, innovative, self-motivated, stimulating, and a good leader (like Bill Clinton). On the bad side, the driven person is cold-blooded and manipulative, unempathetic, impatient, and has a dominating personality. That's enough to send some back to the drawing board.[3]

While these are general personality traits and each person won't fit the description completely, we have seen that every personality type has some attractive and repulsive elements that become very important once the romance cools. The healthy dater takes this phenomenon into account as he decides to commit himself to one person. The healthy man will date women from all four general personality types and combinations (like an expressive-driven person). The idea is to discover which personality style meshes best with his own personality style. There is no one-size-fits-all approach to healthy dating. The healthy man will not delude himself like the mirage man, who enters each relationship thinking he has found the perfect girl. The healthy man, grounded in reality, accepts the good personality traits with the bad. As communication specialist and author Lillian Glass observed, "You can't change people, but you can change your behavior and give them insight into the way they behave towards you."[4] Then, when the healthy man commits to a woman, it is an unconditional love of the whole person, not just her good side.

The healthy man must date with intelligence to find compatibility. He must date to be vulnerable, so the woman can see his true personality traits also. This is the most difficult step in the transition of a mirage man to a healthy man. The healthy man will learn to take risks in dating. He will pursue his relationships in honesty. This allows the woman the rare privilege of choosing or rejecting his true self as her life partner, instead of choosing a mirage. It is hard to believe, but that is what American men routinely did a hundred years ago. Yet today's generation of American men have been taught that this honest behavior is unthinkable.

Candor in dating isn't easy. Even the burliest football player cowers at the notion of risking rejection in dating, but that is the challenge one must take to have a healthy union. Instead of using approval seeking to continue the momentum of the incipient relationship, the healthy man will use the dating process to determine if two people of compatible temperaments also have a core of shared interests. The bottom line of successful dating is: Would you be friends who genuinely enjoy each other's company? Do you share enough common values and goals to survive the long haul of life together? Do you share enough common interests that you would want to spend your precious free time together once the sex gets old? These are the difficult questions that must be answered in the cold light of day if a man wants to break out of the cycle.

A great cinematic example of the correct way to pursue marriage comes from an unlikely source. Alfred Hitchcock, the master of the macabre, crafted a classic movie, *Rear Window*, which deplored the results of the Tiger Woods Syndrome and illustrated how to avoid it. This movie featured James Stewart as Jeff, a lower-class photojournalist, and Grace Kelly as Lisa, an upper-class fashion designer. Jeff breaks his leg and, while laid up in his apartment complex, observes several couples across the courtyard. These couples represent several different types of marriages: both the Tiger Woods Syndrome and the healthy companionate marriage. Professor Virginia Wright Wexman summarizes the courtyard complex:

. . . the newly wedded husband who loses his job because his sexually voracious wife has exhausted him suggests that *marriages should involve satisfactions beyond erotic ones.* The attraction between Miss Lonelyhearts and her composer-neighbor suggests the importance of similar interests as well as sexual rapport in romantic *attachments* and the reunion of Miss Torso and her sailor-husband suggest that marital fulfillment need not necessarily be founded on an attraction to a mate whose appearance conforms to culturally constructed criteria for erotic desirability. The older couple who sleep on the fire escape are posed as people who have reached a stage of marital relations at which sexuality has ceased to be a significant issue; instead, the *complementary and mutually supportive roles* they enact in relation to their little dog hint at the shared parental responsibilities that are conceived as part of the companionate model. Finally, Thorwald, the murderer, may be understood in terms of the desperate lengths to which a husband may be driven if he forms a marriage alliance with a wife who is *not compatible.* (Italics are authors' emphasis.)[5]

In *Rear Window*, Hitchcock shows that artificial intimacy and approval seeking leads to unhappiness. Alfred Hitchcock uses Jeff and Lisa to show us how a healthy relationship can be achieved. Their central conflict is not about sexual attraction and charm but compatibility. Their task is to determine if they possess enough similar interests, values, and goals to share a life together. They must also decide if their personality types are compatible. Finally, can they flesh out complementary and supporting roles as a couple? This is a judgment that must be made with minds cleared from the intoxicating fumes of infatuation. Hitchcock's wonderful examples from across the courtyard are a sharp reminder that the disciplined decision can spare one from a doomed mirage relationship.

Let us now look at a real-life example of a couple that found the way to healthy dating and marriage.

CASE STUDY OF A HEALTHY RELATIONSHIP: BILL AND ELLEN

There are men in America who are not deceptive. They have a clear idea of who they are and what they want in life. They are an endangered species in America today. Bill, a twenty-two-year-old senior history major, lived the values discussed in this book. He entered college three years earlier as the rarest of college freshmen, the type that had already scouted out the university scene and decided exactly what academic and extracurricular activities he would participate in without overdoing it. He brought a similar logic to his dating. He had high visibility as a yell leader, campus political leader, trumpet player in the marching band, and fraternity member. He used his ample connections in all four social circles to survey a wide variety of women. Unlike the rest of his fraternity brothers, he didn't seem driven to have one long-term steady girlfriend. He kept himself commitment free so that he could use the rare opportunity college affords to meet a cross-section of women from across the state. Bill developed a healthy relationship his senior year that led to marriage and family.

Ellen seemed incompatible to Bill at first glance. While Bill was the expressive yell-leader type, the analytical Ellen would stand back out of the glare of the klieg lights and let him drink in the attention. She was not threatened by his celebrity status and his extroverted need to dominate the social scene. He was comfortable being himself and didn't tone it down to please Ellen. She was given the opportunity to accept or reject the real Bill, knowing he would always be the life of the party.

Bill had learned that he didn't get along with the fellow extroverts he had dated. Instead of enjoying each other, he would end up competing with them for the spotlight. For Bill, compatibility in a mate meant he needed an introvert, someone who could appreciate his theatrical talents.

In addition to compatible temperaments, Bill and Ellen shared a core of common interests, including worldview, politics, sports, and religion. They seemed different from the typical college couples of that era who soared like meteors across the summer night sky, only to burn out after a burst of honeymoon glory. Bill and Ellen enjoyed the rarest of gems: a healthy courtship. It was a revolutionary relationship.

LIVING THE HEALTHY RELATIONSHIP

Once the dating relationship grows and deepens in intimacy, the healthy man is faced with the mirage man's dilemma: do I have time in my busy life for a full-time commitment to a woman and my friends? If the healthy man is to keep his life in balance, he must make his close male friendships a priority. Relationships with other men enable him to express feelings and share common interests that have always been an important part of his life. By nurturing these friendships through the development of a new romance, the healthy man will retain trusted confidants with whom to share his ups and downs and gain valuable feedback from a distinctly male perspective.

How revolutionary this concept seems today. But it is nothing new. Historian Ellen Rothman notes that even engaged couples in the 1800s remained socially active with both men and women.[6] Again, the idea was to maintain balance in one's life even as one attained marriage. There never was this artificial isolation leading to a honeymoon. In fact, the honeymoon, which developed in the 1830s and eventually became an American wedding tradition, was originally a bridal trip that included friends and close relatives.[7] Today's honeymoon, where the couple rushes off to a secret, exotic locale isolated from friends and family, is a mutation of the original healthy community celebration of marriage.

When the relationship is built on a foundation of honesty, the woman in the healthy relationship will already know what her man and his friends are really like. She will not view them as a threat but as an important part of her lover's life. The man's friends will likewise affirm the value of the man's new love interest. The inevitable jealousy between the woman and the friends is thus eliminated. Instead of viewing each other with smoldering resentment, the healthy man's friends and his girlfriend will be able to enjoy one another's company. After all, they have much in common—they both care deeply about the healthy man.

By instituting these principles of healthy relating, the honeymoon stage is completely eliminated. Some of you may be disappointed with this statement. We have been conditioned by the media to look forward to this stage like a child looks forward to Christmas or Hanukkah. But the truth is that the honeymoon stage is a monument to the dishonesty of men to women in courtship. The honeymoon is an illusion of love, fueled by the deceptive use of artificial intimacy and approval seeking.

In this stage both partners are loving ephemeral images of each other that will die with the fall leaves. By bypassing the exhausting deceptive game of pretending to be Mr. Sensitive, the healthy man will end up with someone who has chosen him with all of his imperfections. In sharp contrast to the mirage man, he will end up with a woman whom he can truly love and who will love his true self. The relationship will deepen in intimacy as the healthy man practices the lost American art of courtship and marriage.

Consider two simple steps suggested by therapist and

author Marvin Allen: (1) say how you feel, and (2) state what you want. In other words, let your partner know how you're feeling, then tell her what you want or need. "I'm angry that you accepted the dinner invitation without talking to me first. I'd appreciate it if you'd ask me first before you accept."[8] By dealing with conflict in this open, honest way, anger is dealt with immediately and is not allowed to internalize into resentment. The woman will be able to deal with the man's needs instead of spending hours, days, or years trying to figure out her mate's frozen feelings. As stated in countless women's magazines, the woman will be enjoying what she has always dreamed of in a marriage: intimacy. She will feel good about her relationship, and so will he!

This is the good news offering the possibility of a high level of happiness in marriage. American men once practiced such healthy courtship and marriage behavior, so we know it is possible to get back to this marital garden. We're hoping that the ideas presented in this book will be the beginning of an awakening in America. The alienation of men and women is not a permanent condition we must accept as normal. Each of us must take that first step toward honesty and health to break the deceptive chain of relationship and societal death.

❧ NOTES ❧

Chapter 1

1 Abcarian, Robin. "Happily Married . . . or Just Nuts?" *Los Angeles Times,* July 23, 1995, sec. E, 1, 4.

Chapter 3

1 Rothman, Ellen K. *Hands and Hearts: A History of Courtship in America.* New York: Basic Books, 1984, 103.

2 Wexman, Virginia Wright. *Creating the Couple: Love, Marriage, and the Hollywood Performance.* New Jersey: Princeton University Press, 1993, 12.

3 Sollors, Werner. *Beyond Ethnicity: Consent and Descent in American Culture.* Oxford: Oxford University Press, 1986, 12.

4 Wexman, Virginia Wright. *Creating the Couple: Love, Marriage, and the Hollywood Performance.* New Jersey: Princeton University Press, 1993, 13.

5 Rothman, Ellen K. *Hands and Hearts: A History of Courtship in America.* New York: Basic Books, 1984, 68, 73.

6 Wexman, Virginia Wright. *Creating the Couple: Love, Marriage, and the Hollywood Performance.* New Jersey: Princeton University Press, 1993, 13.

7 Wexman, Virginia Wright. *Creating the Couple: Love, Marriage, and the Hollywood Performance.* New Jersey: Princeton University Press, 1993, 170.

8. Wexman, Virginia Wright. *Creating the Couple: Love, Marriage, and the Hollywood Performance.* New Jersey: Princeton University Press, 1993, 274

9. Charen, Mona. "Divorce Can't Be Labeled As No One's Fault." *Daily News* 15 February 1996, News: 23.

10 Due, Tananarive. "Sometimes, No Choice Beats Too Much Choice." *Daily News* 22 February 1996, L.A. Life.

11 Rothman, Ellen K. *Hands and Hearts: A History of Courtship in America.* New York: Basic Books, 1984, 109.

12 Rothman, Ellen K. *Hands and Hearts: A History of Courtship in America.* New York: Basic Books, 1984, 192.

13 Rothman, Ellen K. *Hands and Hearts: A History of Courtship in America.* New York: Basic Books, 1984, 224–225.

14 Johnson, Reed. "Sinatra—Other Than His Way." *Daily News* 6 January 1998, L.A. Life 3.

15 Whitehead, Barbara Defoe. "Families, Race, Poverty and Welfare." *Daily News* (Los Angeles) January 1, 1995, Viewpoint section 1.

16 Medved, Michael. *Hollywood vs. America.* New York: Harper Collins, 1992.

17 Rochlin, Margy. "George Clooney." *U.S. Magazine,* July 1997: 56.

18 Jayson, Sharon. "Divorce Declining But So Is Marriage," *USA Today,* July 18, 2005: 3A.

19 Popenoe, David and Barbara Dafoe Whitehead. "The National Marriage Project." January 1999, smartmarriage.com/cohabit.html.

20 Wetzstein, Cheryl. "Unwed Couples, At 4.1 Million, Still On the Rise Nationally." *The Washington Times,* 31 August 1993: 1.

21 "Girl Meets Boy," *Wall Street Journal,* August 3, 1001: A6.

22 Glenn, Norval, and Elisabeth Marquardt. Hooking Up, Hanging Out, and Hoping for Mr. Right. Institute for American Values Report to Independent Women's Forum, 2001.

Chapter 4

1 Forward, Susan. *Men Who Hate Women and the Women Who Love Them.* New York: Bantam, 2002.

2 CBS News. "Tiger Texts Show Weakness for Woman." December 10, 2009, www.cbsnews.com/stories/2009/12/10/.../main5961619.shtml.

Chapter 5

1 Gold, Todd. "Crazy Love." *US Weekly,* 26 June 2000:58.

2 Allen, Woody, dir. *Annie Hall,* 1977. Videocassette.

3 De Turenne, Veronique. "Love at First Sight." *Daily News* (Los Angeles), February 13, 1995, L.A. Life sec., 7.

4 Kazanjian, Dodie. "An Artful Existence." *Vogue,* 1998, 146.

5 Duffy, Karen. "Breakup With Moore Has Willis Very Sad." *Daily News*, 26 June 1998:N2.

6 Gold, Todd. "Crazy Love." *US Weekly*, 26 June 2000:58.

7 Adler, Eric. "Deception Finds Its Way into Marriage." *Daily New* (Los Angeles), August 22, 1994, L.A. Life sec., 8.

8 Gregory, Kim Lamb. "Life's a Love Song, for Old, Young Alike." *Ventura County Star*, April 22, 1998, sec. C, 8.

9 De Turenne, Veronique. "Love at First Sight." *Daily News* (Los Angeles), February 13, 1995, L.A. Life sec., 7.

10 Morse, Steve. "Simon Muses About Former Lost Loves in Melodic 'Letters Never Sent.'" *Daily News*, November 20, 1994, L.A. Life sec., 11.

11 Street, Morris. "What Men Will Never Tell You." *Ladies Home Journal*, April 1994, 106, 209.

Chapter 6

1 *Late Show with David Letterman*. Interview with Alec Baldwin, June 27, 1994.

2 Smolowe, Jill. "Star Blight." *People*, April 17, 2000, 98.

3 Sondheimer, Eric. "Behind Every Great Man." *Daily News*, 18 September 1996, Sports: 3.

4 Associated Press. "Marriage Too Breathtaking." *Daily News* (Los Angeles), February 20, 1996, news sec., 6.

5 Beck, Marilyn, and Stacy Jenel Smith. "Will Twin Cousins Laugh Alike, Walk Alike Again?" *Daily News* (Los Angeles), October 11, 1996, L.A. Life sec., 17.

6 Associated Press. "Marriage Too Breathtaking." *Daily News* (Los Angeles), February 20, 1996, news sec., 6.

7 Adler, Eric. "Deception Finds Its Way into Marriage." *Daily News* (Los Angeles), August 22, 1994, L.A. Life sec., 8.

8 Eveld, Edward M. "Author Suggests Men Cloak Their Unhappiness in Aloof Attitudes." *Daily News* (Los Angeles), March 12, 1998, L.A. Life sec., 9.

9 Means, Patrick. "Men's Issues: Making It Through the Minefields." *Steps*, Summer 1994, 13.

10 Allen, Marvin. *Angry Men, Passive Men*. New York: Fawcett Columbine Books, 1993, 15.

11 Rosenthal, Phil. "Mrs. B's Hubby Facing the Music." *Daily News* (Los Angeles), September 27, 1995, L.A. Life sec., 3.

12 Lieblich, Julia. "Unequally Yoked." *Ventura County Star,* October 11, 1997, sec. C, 1.

13 Adler, Eric. "Deception Finds Its Way into Marriage." *Daily News* (Los Angeles), August 22, 1994, L.A. Life sec., 8.

Chapter 7

1 De Witt, Barbara. "Finding Love that Will Last." *Daily News* (Los Angeles), February 16, 1995, L.A. Life sec., 8.

2 Duffy, Karen. "Kuralt's Mistress Is Off the Road in His Will." *Daily News* (Los Angeles), May 27, 1998.

3 Associated Press. "Two–timer Charged with Killing Three." *Ventura County Star,* October 11, 1997, sec. B, 11.

4 Allen, Marvin. *Angry Men Passive Men.* New York: Fawcett Columbine Books, 1993, 157.

5 Vinnedge, Mary. "Different Desires for Single Seniors." *Daily News,* 10 December 1996: LA Life 10.

6 Ackerman, Robert. *Silent Sons.* New York: Simon and Schuster, 1993.

Chapter 8

1 Mellen, Joan. *Big Bad Wolves: Masculinity in the American Film.* New York: Pantheon Books, 1997, 14–15.

2 Hendrix, Harvey. *Getting the Love You Want.* New York: Harper Perennial, 1998, 53.

Chapter 9

1 Duffy, Karen. "Breakup with Moore Has Willis Very Sad." *Daily News* (Los Angeles), February 22, 1996: LA Life N 2.

2 Associated Press "How to Stop Falling Out of Love, into Rut of Silent Boredom," *Daily News* (Los Angeles), November 5, 1996. Life Section, 10.

3 Dorman, Lesley. "What Are You Thinking?" *Redbook,* April 1994, 94–97.

4 Blowen, Michael. "Memories Are Made of This." *Daily News* (Los Angeles), December 28, 1995, LA Life Section, 3.

5 Allen, Marvin. *Angry Men, Passive Men.* New York: Fawcett Columbine Books, 1993, 101.

6 Rhodes, Sonya. "The Sex Game That Can Ruin a Good Marriage." *McCall's,* July 1993, 67–69.

7 Street, Morris. "What Men Will Never Tell You." *Ladies Home Journal,* April 1994, 106, 209.

8 Gray, John, Ph.D. "Great Unmarried Sex." *Ladies Home Journal,* May 1995, 86.

9 Allen, Marvin. *Angry Men, Passive Men.* New York: Fawcett Columbine Books, 1993, 101, 102

10 Schwartz, Pepper. "Sexless Marriages Survive But Don't Thrive." *Daily News* (Los Angeles), January 30, 1996, LA Life Section, 7.

11 Adler, Eric. "Deception Finds Its Way into Marriage." *Daily News* (Los Angeles), August 22, 1994, LA Life Section, 8.

12 Allen, Marvin. *Angry Men, Passive Men.* New York: Fawcett Columbine Books, 1993, 102

13 May, Gerald. *Addiction and Grace.* San Francisco: Harper One, 1988, 38–39.

14 Duffy, Karen. "Bridges' Writer's Marriage Is Over." *Daily News* (Los Angeles), June 26, 1998, News Section, 2.

15 Harley, Willard F. "Why Women Leave Men." *New Man,* August 1998:68.

16 Dobson, James. "Opening the Trap Door." *Daily News* (Los Angeles), September 1995, Section 4.

17 Gardner, Elysa. "Ditching the Love Circus." *Los Angeles Times,* September 22, 1996, Calendar, 62.

Chapter 12

1 About.com: Marriage. "Tiger Woods and Elin Nordegren Marriage Profile, January 31, 2010, http://marriage.about.com/cs/celebritymarriages/p/tigerwoods.htm.

2 Friends in Recovery. *The Twelve Steps: A Spiritual Journey.* San Diego, CA: Recovery Publications, 1988.

3 Landers, Ann. "Widow Aghast at Her Husband's Secret Side." *Daily News* (Los Angeles), December 18, 1995, L.A. Life sec., 16.

4 Street, Morris. "What Men Will Never Tell You." *Ladies Home Journal,* April 1994, 106, 209.

Chapter 13

1 Morrow, Lance. "Are Men Really That Bad?" *Time,* 14 February 1994: 52–59.

2 Allen, Marvin. *Angry Men, Passive Men.* New York: Fawcett Columbine Books, 1993, 98.

3 Haas, Jane Glenn. "Separate Beds Needn't Mean Separate Lives." *Daily News* 29 October 1996, L.A. Life: 10.

Chapter 14

1 Rothman, Ellen K. *Hands and Hearts: A History of Courtship in America.* New York: Basic Books, 1984.
2 Strauss, Bob. "Chutzpah Halle: Changes On and Off the Screen." *Daily News (Los Angeles)*, March 28, 1997, L.A. Life weekend sec., 3.
3 Merrill, David. "Personality Styles and Effective Performance." Boca Raton, FL: CRC Press LLC, 1999.
4 Weldon, Michele. "Ways to Make Bad Relationships Get Better." *Daily News* 5 February 1997, LA Life, 9.
5 Wexman, Virginia Wright. *Creating the Couple: Love, Marriage, and the Hollywood Performance.* New Jersey: Princeton University Press, 1993.
6 Rothman, Ellen K. *Hands and Hearts: A History of Courtship in America.* New York: Basic Books, 1984, 162.
7 Rothman, Ellen K. *Hands and Hearts: A History of Courtship in America.* New York: Basic Books, 1984, 82.
8 Allen, Marvin. *Angry Men, Passive Men.* New York: Fawcett Columbine Books, 1993, 176.

INDEX

Page numbers followed by an *f* indicate figures.

༻ ABOUT THE AUTHORS ༺

J. R. Bruns, M.D., is a psychiatrist and medical director of La Mer Integrative & Behavioral Medical Group. After earning his Bachelor of Arts in Pharmacology at UCSB, he obtained his medical degree at Case Western School of Medicine. Following the completion of his psychiatric residency at USC, he was an assistant clinical professor. Dr. Bruns is a noted speaker, lecturer, and expert on a wide variety of personality issues, including anxiety disorders, social phobias, and behavioral disorders. He and his wife Jeanne have been married for thirty-seven years, raised three children, and currently reside in southern California.

R. A. Richards II has a Bachelor of Arts degree in Communication Studies from UCLA. In addition to studying interpersonal and mass communications, he honed his skills in evaluating information from a life sciences curriculum and earned a Doctorate in Dental Surgery from Northwestern University. Dr. Richards served as a moderator and small group facilitator for a twelve-step group for codependency.

Visit: www.tigerwoods-syndrome.com.